Contents

About the Authors

Jon Paxman

Jon joined 2020health in 2011, transferring his writing, editing and research skills from the worlds of media and classical music. He has contributed to a number of health IT reports, including 'Personal Health Records: Putting patients in Control?' and 2020health's independent evaluation of the 'Yorkshire and the Humber Regional Telehealth Hub'. More recently he co-authored 'Making Connections', a report preparing for a transatlantic exchange between the US VHA and England's NHS to support the adoption of digital health. Jon was project lead on 'Personal Health Budgets: a revolution in personalisation' (2013) and is currently involved on a second report for 2020health's 'Fit for School' workstream, exploring ways of improving the health and wellbeing of school pupils and staff.

Gail Beer
Director of Operations
2020health

Gail worked in the NHS for over 30 years, latterly as an Executive Director at Barts and the London NHS Trust. She trained as a general nurse at St Bartholomew's Hospital before undertaking a course in Renal Nursing at the Royal Free Hospital. After a number of senior nursing posts within London she moved into management, taking a Masters in Health Management at City University, before becoming Director of Operations at BLT. Since leaving Barts and the London NHS Trust she has worked as an independent consultant in healthcare. Gail was a member of the team that produced the Independent Review of NHS and Social Care IT, commissioned by Stephen O'Brien MP. Gail's main interests are in creating a society that values the contribution older people make, compassion in caring and preventing disease caused by poor lifestyle choices.

1. Executive Summary

1.1 Background

Vaccination ranks only below clean water as the most important health intervention in the world for saving lives and promoting good health. England's Childhood Immunisation Programme (CIP) currently delivers routine vaccinations for 12 infectious diseases: most vaccinations are administered in four stages to infants from two to thirteen months, with flu vaccine (nasal spray) given to children aged two and three, and two pre-school injections (DTaP/IPV booster and MMR second dose) given at three years and four months, or soon after.

Enormous improvements in uptake have been seen in recent years, with a greater proportion of children vaccinated now than ever before. The gains have been realised through a multi-strategic approach, focusing on improvements to IT systems and data accuracy, access to services, public awareness and catch-up campaigns. Gains from 2006/7 to 2012/13 include the three-in-one Measles, Mumps and Rubella first dose (MMR1) vaccine, with national coverage rising from 85% to 92%, and the DTaP/IPV booster, rising from 79% to 89%. Almost every locality in England has seen year-on-year gains since 2007: those working in immunisation have a right to be proud of their achievements.

So why have we written this report?

Firstly, the CIP is facing challenges following the reorganisation of NHS commissioning structures, introduced April 2013. Key concerns include: confusion around accountability pathways, particularly at the local level; a lack of clarity as to who is responsible for the funding of immunisation training; and incomplete recruitment of Screening and Immunisation Teams. According to a number of experts we interviewed, the new CIP structures have also left many providers at a loss as to how to access expert immunisation advice. It was their considered opinion that staff confidence, key to the success of the CIP, has declined. Further, a certain amount of local expertise has been lost to the system through the decommissioning of district immunisation coordinator posts. While some immunisation coordinators remain (funded by community trusts, for example), there appears to be reduced capacity to deliver training and support.

Secondly, no Local Authority in England, even after the gains of recent years, can claim 'herd immunity' for children across the full range of infectious diseases targeted by the CIP. For example, herd immunity to measles requires sustained ≥95% vaccination uptake in each and every district. And if MMR coverage of around 92% sounds impressive, we need look no further than Wales 2012/13 for the impact of sub-optimal uptake – generally implying anything below 95%. Wales had seen three consecutive years (since quarter 3, 2009) with MMR1 uptake between 92% and 94% at 2 years, only to then see their one to four year-olds as one of the worst affected age groups during the measles outbreak. Measles cases among the unvaccinated (all ages) outnumbered those vaccinated by more than 95:1. Wales is a salutary reminder of why the CIP has to aim for 100%, even though this figure is almost certainly never achievable.

Thirdly, there is still substantial variation of uptake within England and thousands of children remain exposed to vaccine-preventable diseases. The CIP is not yet a truly equitable system. Variation of uptake is particularly pronounced in London and Birmingham, and more generally across the South East of England. Other localities may be reporting generally high uptake, but still seeing worrying internal variation at the district level. Lower uptake, as we explore in Section 3, is often linked to a complex interaction of social factors, exacerbated by the lack of easy access to services.

1. Executive Summary

The following key recommendations are designed to support increased uptake and reduced health inequalities in the CIP. Numbers in brackets correspond to the order in which these recommendations appear throughout the report. There are a number of supporting recommendations which have not been included in the executive summary.

1.2 National Level Action

Recommendations: CIP delivery and support	Action to be taken by:
(1,3) The DH should tackle the perceived lack of 'system ownership' by identifying clear pathways of accountability: locally, sub-regionally (e.g. Area Teams) and regionally. This includes making clear the role and expectations of public health teams in Local Authorities, and CCGs in their 'duty of quality improvement'.	Department of Health (DH)
(6) Commissioning responsibilities around immunisation training need to be clearly defined. This should include guidance to General Practice as to whether it is responsible for any funding of training.	NHS England
(8) The DH should consider a national immunisation advice line for health care professionals, staffed by experts but also with wide online functionality, so to make immunisation advice readily accessible to providers in both urban and remote regions.	DH
(9) Immunisation, as part of the Healthy Child Programme, should be a mandatory component of Health Visitor training so to maximise opportunities for access to services. HV delivery of immunisation should only occur where parents are considered unlikely to attend GP settings or child health clinics – thus as a last resort.	DH Public Health England (PHE)

Recommendations: GP DES payments	Action to be taken by:
(10) (General) DES payments for the CIP should be revised with raised thresholds.	DH, in consultation with: NHS England PHE
(11) (Specific) The lowest DES threshold should be raised from 70% to 80%. We also recommend a three-tier DES system that incentivises optimal uptake, with a new 95% reward facilitated through a reduction of the 90% payment; the relative scale of financial reward thus rising: 1 (80%): 2.5 (90%): 3.5 (95%).	DH, in consultation with: NHS England PHE
(12) Public health and General Practice need to be focused on the same targets. DES payments should therefore be aligned to Child Health Information System data and the COVER schedule to encourage General Practice in timely immunisation and reporting.	DH

Recommendation: IT solutions	Action to be taken by:
(13) Most children born in England have a Summary Care Record (SCR) created at birth. The electronic SCR should be promoted from the outset as a record for CIP activity, with immunisation status included as SCR 'core data'.	DH

1.3 Local Level Action

Recommendations: Access / IT solutions	Action to be taken by:
(15) An 'Area Immunisation Task Force' should be considered for each Area to deliver mobile immunisation services to the 'hard-to-reach', as well as run community immunisation clinics in localities that lack capacity for such services.	NHS England Public Health Screening and Immunisation Area teams
(16) NHS England (currently responsible for commissioning CHIS systems) needs to review its provision for routine CHIS data cleansing and gleaning, and recognise this as a priority for all Child Health Departments. This vital procedure is not yet embedded across England.	NHS England LA Public Health

Recommendations: catch-up / public information	Action to be taken by:
(18) Learning from successful, cost-effective catch-up strategies needs much better dissemination. Rarely are these initiatives written up with robust data and very few have been published in the public domain.	LA Public Health DH
(19) District-level, if not borough-wide, 'fit-for-school' immunisation advertising campaigns should be considered, maximising transport-network and shop-window opportunities to warn at-risk populations of the dangers of missed vaccinations. It should be recognised that local Public Health is often eligible for discounted advertising rates.	LA Public Health CCGs

Other recommendations:	Action to be taken by:
(20) The assessment of immunisation status needs to become a core area of the School Entry Health Check for all children. Nurses need to take this opportunity to promote the importance of vaccination and help arrange catch-up where necessary.	PHE LA Public Health
(21) NHS England, working with local Public Health, should consider recruiting key workers (such as community health trainers) from minority communities to act as trusted immunisation champions. Such health workers could operate at an Area-wide level if necessary.	NHS England LA Public Health
(23) The use of text technology needs to be actively promoted among General Practice, so to facilitate efficient appointment call and timely reminders, reducing both paperwork and DNA rates.	Screening and Immunisation Teams CCGs

1.4 Conclusion

Some of the above recommendations build on existing strategies, others suggest changes or new agencies of support. None are designed to dismantle the new CIP architecture. It is essential that the new system is allowed time to embed. But it is also clear that a multi-strategic approach is required to make significant progress towards increased uptake and equity within the CIP. It is therefore important that immunisation is given due priority both at the 'area' level and at the local level, by Public Health, CCGs and Health and Wellbeing Boards. The danger is to see the CIP on a safe trajectory towards improvement on the basis of legacy PCT strategies. But with key changes to governance and commissioning models, now is the time to take stock and recalibrate the CIP, most importantly ensuring that even hard to reach children have easy access to services, giving them the greatest chance of maximum protection from communicable diseases.

2. Introduction

England boasts a world-class Childhood Immunisation Programme (CIP). The CIP currently delivers routine vaccinations for 12 infectious diseases: most vaccinations are administered in four stages to infants from two to thirteen months, with flu vaccine (nasal spray) given to children aged two and three, and two pre-school injections (DTaP/IPV booster and MMR second dose) given at three years and four months, or soon after.

The two public health interventions that have had the greatest impact on the world's health are clean water and vaccines.

World Health Organisation

Though trailing the UK's devolved nations in uptake, England has seen significant improvements across the CIP during the last few years thanks to increased investment in catch-up campaigns, widening of access to services, IT solutions and robust data cleansing. Notable gains from 2006/7 to 2012/13 include the three-in-one Measles, Mumps and Rubella first dose (MMR1) vaccine,[1] with national coverage rising from 85% to 92%, and the DTaP/IPV booster, rising from 79% to 89%. Other gains for the period have been of lower increments, but still encouraging, such as MenC coverage at 12 months rising from 91% to 95%. Five-in-one (DTaP/IPV/Hib) coverage at 24 months stood at 96% in 2012/13.

COVER statistics suggest that in many places across England pre-school populations are benefitting from 'herd immunity' to certain diseases. But due to variation of uptake over recent years, and the variation that exists at the local district level, no Local Authority can claim herd immunity for all children across the full range of infectious diseases targeted by the CIP.

If uptake of around 92% sounds impressive, it falls short of herd immunity to a disease such as measles, as the 2012/13 outbreak in Wales demonstrated. Wales had seen three consecutive years with MMR1 uptake between 92% and 94% at two years of age,[2] only to then see their one to four year-olds as one of the worst affected age groups during the measles outbreak. Measles cases among the unvaccinated (all ages) vastly outnumbered those of vaccinated individuals. In April 2013 Public Services for Wales reported: 'emerging data suggests that in the outbreak area one dose of MMR vaccine protects against measles in more than 95 out of every 100 vaccinated,[3] and two doses protects in around 99 out of every 100 vaccinated.' To argue the case for both the importance of herd immunity levels and the efficacy of the MMR vaccine, we need look no further than Wales 2012/13 (see also Appendix B).

Raising uptake must remain a priority for England's Childhood Immunisation Programme, with concerted effort to address the variation of uptake itself. The CIP at this present time is far from an equitable system; its weaknesses are most pronounced among mobile populations (e.g. recent immigrants and traveller communities) and vulnerable children, the latter often resident in care and foster homes and frequently moved to new localities for reasons of safety.

Added to these concerns are the considerable challenges facing the CIP following the reorganisation of NHS commissioning structures, instituted April 2013. We have heard opinion from a number of immunisation experts that the CIP is experiencing instability, with many immunisation staff confused within the new system and uncertain in matters of training and advice. Staff confidence – noted in JSNA

---

1. Reports, publicity and workshops around the discrediting of the MMR-autism link has undoubtedly helped increase MMR uptake.
2. Uptake for Wales in quarter 3, 2009, stood at 91.9% for MMR1; uptake by quarter 3, 2012, had risen to 94%. Source: National Public Services for Wales.
3. http://www.wales.nhs.uk/sitesplus/888/page/66389#d Accessed 26.11.2013

guidelines as key to the success of the CIP – has declined. Moreover, local expertise has been lost to the system, with many posts of immunisation coordinator abolished and, according to some we interviewed, reduced capacity on the ground to deliver domiciliary visits and catch-up interventions.[4]

Given the logistical challenges of reaching diverse and often mobile populations, compounded by confusion amongst many working within the system, how does the CIP move forward and build on the successes of recent years? Is best practice, as understood pre-NHS reforms, still relevant and/or achievable? This report takes a timely look at these pressing concerns and presents recommendations applicable to both the short and long term.

2.1 Process adopted

This project was undertaken between May and November 2013. A Steering Group of unpaid experts was convened to help focus direction, raise questions, guide research and scrutinise findings as the project progressed.

Literature review: we conducted a wide-ranging review of published research and opinion online, principally from the UK but also from other European countries and the USA. From UK sources we have assembled recent data around vaccination coverage and population demographics, and accessed reports on best practice and catch-up strategies of the last five years.

It is important to note that during the project research period we found little published material pertaining to the new immunisation landscape (that is, post April 2013), including experience of the new CIP support structures and commissioning processes.

Interviews: we conducted 14 semi-structured interviews between August and October 2013 with experts working at various levels of immunisation. Most were local staff involved in supporting the CIP – immunisation specialist nurses, consultant paediatricians and local authority public health staff. Interviewees were asked to share opinions on best practice and transferrable learning for the CIP, taking into account opportunities or challenges under the new NHS structures. They were also asked to share their on-the-ground experience of immunisation post-April 2013. This included reports on the experience of general practice as the principal providers of the CIP.[5] Our interviews were largely London-focused, involving representatives from ten boroughs.

Informal contacts: further evidence and opinion was gathered via informal communication (by phone or email) with local authorities in and outside of London.

Workshop: 2020health held a CIP workshop on 9 September, 2013, at which we presented various statements and questions arising from our interviews up to that time. The workshop was attended by a broad range of experts from Public Health England, NHS England and the National Institute for Health and Clinical Excellence (NICE); also attending were immunisation specialist nurses, health visitor and school nurse team leaders, experts in paediatric immunology and paediatric intensive care, and representatives from the Royal College of Nursing and the Royal College of Paediatricians and Child Health. Sponsor representatives from Pfizer attended in an observational capacity only.

A full list of interviewees, workshop attendees and steering group members is provided in Appendix A.

---

4.   2020health interviews, August – October, 2013.
5.   Limitations of scope did not allow us to conduct interviews with immunisation providers in general practice.

2.2 Report structure

This report is split into two principal sections: the first sets context; the second identifies key problems and solutions.

Context sections

Section 3:   highlighting inequalities of coverage in England's Childhood Immunisation Programme
Section 4:   identifying the new key CIP delivery structures, while also noting the unanswered questions around delivery and accountability

Solutions sections

Section 5:   considering important issues at the national level, and identifying potential solutions
Section 6:   considering important issues at the local level, and identifying potential solutions

Section 7:   conclusion

Many of the solutions presented in this report derive from collective (but not in every case unanimous) opinion, generated by professionals in interview and at our workshop.

3. CIP variation in England: a snapshot of inequalities

Few words carry more importance to the NHS as 'equality' and 'equity'. In healthcare, equality means treating each person as equally important and ensuring equal access, while equity means meeting the needs of each individual, which may be different (therefore not 'equal') from one to the next. In terms of prevention, immunisation is the only area of healthcare delivery considered essential for all children: [6] it is therefore one of the most important services in which to strive for the very highest standards of equality and equity.

Immunisation coverage in England has improved dramatically over recent years thanks to increased investment and activity around data management, IT solutions, access and catch-up strategies. And yet, despite commendable success, there still remains both shortfall and considerable variation in coverage across England. Tens of thousands of children in England are not being immunised, or sufficiently immunised, year on year. As of early 2013, PCTs in the north of England had achieved highest uptake in general, though even there, few had reached 'herd immunity' levels across the full CIP. Those levels vary according to disease, with the most infectious, measles, requiring at least 95% coverage (MMR first dose by 24 months, second dose by age 5).[7] The cumulative effect of sub-optimal immunisation (year after year) means most localities in England have thousands of young children at risk from one or more infectious diseases.

In most circumstances, the sensible public health practice is to aim for 100% coverage, with all the doses recommended, recognising that 100% is never achievable.

Oxford Journals:
Clinical Infectious Diseases, 2011

Table 3a gives indication of the variation of CIP delivery across England, citing areas of high and low uptake in selected regions. It should be borne in mind that COVER data for the fourth quarter will have been collected at a time of system flux, post-April 2013, which may have impacted data accuracy. A counterpart table in Appendix C presents approximate numbers and percentages of unvaccinated children (selected vaccines only) for the same locations, at 24 months & 5 years, for 2012–13.

---

6. Notwithstanding the very few children for whom immunisation is hazardous due to specific existing medical conditions
7. BMJ 2011. Improving MMR vaccination rates: herd immunity is a realistic goal; 343 doi: http://dx.doi.org/10.1136/bmj.d5703 (4 October 2011)

Table 3a: Percentage of children by 12 months, 24 months
& 5 years, selected areas in England. 2012–13

SHA/PCTs	Immunised at 12 months %			Immunised at 24 months %					Immunised at 5th birthday %	
	DTaP/ IPV/Hib	MenC	PCV	DTaP/ IPV/Hib	MenC primary	MMR 1st dose	Hib/ MenC booster	PCV booster	DTaP/ IPV booster	MMR 1st and 2nd dose
England	94.7	93.9	94.4	96.3	95.1	92.3	92.7	92.5	88.9	87.7
North East	96.5	96.0	96.4	97.8	97.0	94.1	95.5	95.0	93.0	91.7
South Tyneside	99.0	98.8	99.0	99.0	98.3	96.6	97.5	97.4	95.0	93.0
Hartlepool	93.9	93.4	93.5	95.2	92.4	89.2	90.7	89.9	96.1	86.9
North West	95.9	95.6	95.8	97.4	95.8	94.9	94.9	94.8	91.3	91.6
Salford	98.4	96.1	96.5	99.0	94.6	98.4	98.3	97.5	97.4	97.0
Manchester	95.7	94.5	95.1	96.3	93.2	92.7	91.3	92.4	94.8	87.2
West Midlands	94.5	94.1	94.1	96.6	96.2	92.7	92.0	93.0	89.4	87.9
Walsall Teaching	97.6	97.4	97.4	98.8	98.6	97.0	96.9	97.5	96.7	95.0
Birmingham East & North	88.9	88.4	88.3	92.8	93.3	85.3	82.7	86.2	81.5	79.6
London	91.1	89.9	90.8	93.6	90.9	87.1	87.3	86.6	79.9	80.8
Tower Hamlets	96.8	95.5	96.0	97.3	93.8	93.8	94.4	93.5	94.4	93.4
Newham	86.4	85.7	85.8	91.0	88.0	82.2	82.0	82.0	67.9	71.9
Westminster*	79.0	75.9	78.7	81.9	76.8	77.4	77.0	75.1	76.6	75.4
South East Coast	93.7	93.1	93.2	95.0	93.7	91.5	91.6	90.9	90.6	85.9
Eastern & Coastal Kent	95.6	95.2	95.4	97.6	96.7	94.7	94.7	95.6	93.9	92.0
Surrey	87.8	87.1	87.2	89.4	87.9	83.6	83.8	84.3	87.0	76.4

* Uptake may be higher than reported due to possible lack of systematic reporting of immunisation delivered by private practice.

The 2012/13 data quoted show something of the variation of uptake across England, with marked inequalities evident in the West Midlands and South East. Variation in uptake of the pre-school 4-in-1 booster and MMR second dose is above 20% between some struggling London boroughs and the best performing local authorities in England.[8] London also has the most internal variation of uptake of any city: inequalities within the CIP are nowhere more pronounced. Table 3b (pages 15 & 16) brings further focus on London, with a selection of boroughs representing the full gamut of uptake (high, average and low) and with challenges, key demographics and various bespoke interventions listed. It is important to note that even where primary vaccination uptake is reasonably high, pre-school booster and MMR second dose uptake may be relatively poor, leaving many children with sub-optimal protection.

3.1 Who is not being immunised?

In order to develop effective immunisation strategies it is important to recognise exactly who is not being immunised, and why. Research has found that low uptake is conspicuous among vulnerable groups, including (in no particular order):[9]

1. Asylum seekers
2. Homeless families (those housed in temporary accommodation)
3. Looked after children/children in care
4. Children with physical or learning difficulties
5. Children of teenage or lone parents
6. Children not registered with a GP
7. Younger children from large families
8. Children who are hospitalised

Another approach to understanding uptake is presented by the European Centre for Disease Prevention and Control, which cites a range of characteristics for those who do not follow the vaccination programme, in part or full.[10] Four key groups have been identified:

I.   **'The hesitant'** – those who have concerns about perceived safety issues and/or are unsure about needs, procedures and timings for immunising

II.   **'The unconcerned'** – those for whom immunisation is considered a low priority with no real perceived risk of vaccine preventable diseases

III.   **'The poorly reached'** – those with limited or difficult access to services, related to social exclusion, poverty and, in the case of more integrated and affluent populations, factors related to convenience

IV.   **'The active resisters'** – those with personal, cultural or religious beliefs which discourage or exclude vaccination

Both approaches to understanding uptake need to be borne in mind: for example, parents who are asylum seekers, or housed in temporary accommodation, may identify with categories I, II, or IV, even if they fall into category III by default.

---

8.   HSCIC NHS Immunisation Statistics, 2012-13
9.   Islington JSNA 2009/10
10. http://www.ecdc.europa.eu/en/healthtopics/immunisation/comms-aid/Pages/protection.aspx Accessed 2nd October 2013

There is great uncertainty as to the respective proportions of people hesitant, unconcerned or actively resistant to vaccination.[11] 'Active resisters' include some highly educated parents influenced by negative media around vaccination, or those who favour the approach of 'natural' medicines or homeopathy.[12]

A number of those we interviewed for the project felt that the 'active resisters' category had been historically over emphasised due to widespread refusal of MMR following the fallacious scare of 1998.[13] Some felt this had become an excuse for low uptake across the whole CIP. While anecdotal information around vaccine-resisters has been published, we were not able to find any robust quantitative data on the extent of active resistance within England.

3.2 Challenges of high levels of population mobility and ethnic mix
A third category of challenges is created by high levels of population churn and ethnic diversity. Parents may want their children immunised, but are confounded in part by their own transience or language barriers.

In the case of population churn, Public Health relies on robust and efficient information management, so that individuals may be tracked and immunisation data processed easily. In recent years much data processing has become electronic and more efficient, but a great deal of manual management is still required in many localities, complicated by the fact that some GP practices consider immunisation data flow to the Child Health Information System as low priority.

The question of language barriers and communication strategy varies across different areas. Immunisation leaflets in translation are of course an important resource. However it is a challenge to produce literature in all first languages spoken in a particular borough, and little help if members of the target population are illiterate.

3.3 Inequalities: in summary
In England prosperity and deprivation often sit side by side – one can be a five minute walk away from the other. But there should be no 'have' and 'have-nots' in the Childhood Immunisation Programme. Tower Hamlets and Islington have gone some way towards proving that high levels of health equity can be achieved in the CIP in areas where significant deprivation and population mobility exist (see Table 3b). An 'ambition of aspiration', as one of our interviewees put it, needs to be replicated across London, Birmingham and beyond.

The challenge for Public Health is to really know the population: who they are, where they are, their immunisation status and willingness to participate in the CIP. That requires robust data gathering and transfer as part of the long-term strategy. But short-term interventions are often needed also, which may involve additional resources for limited periods.[14]

11. Harrison K, Verma A, Clough G, Morton W, University of Manchester/HPA, 2011. Determinants of MMR uptake
12. NHS Choices: vaccination myths. Accessed 5.11.13. Available: http://www.nhs.uk/Conditions/vaccinations/Pages/myths-truths-kids-vaccines.aspx
13. Mixer R, Jamrozik K, Newsom D. Journal of Epidemiology and Community Health, 2007. Ethnicity as a correlate of the uptake of the first dose of mumps, measles and rubella vaccine.
14. National Institute for Health and Clinical Excellence: Costing statement: Reducing differences in the uptake of immunisation. Available: http://www.nice.org.uk/nicemedia/pdf/PH21CostStatement.pdf

Table 3b: Immunisation inequalities – a snapshot (continued overleaf)

Former PCTs: positioned by imms uptake 2012/13	Years (COVER)	DTaP/ IPV/Hib (primary) % 24 mnths	MenC (primary) % 24 mnths	MMR (1st dose) % 24 mnths	DTaP/IPV Booster % 5th birthday	MMR (1st and 2nd dose) % 5th b'day	Aprx. Pop. turnover (in, out) 2008-09[a]
Tower Hamlets	2007/8	69	69	78	68	66	23%
	2012/13	97	94	94	94	93	
Hillingdon	2007/8	90	87	75	n/a	n/a	14%
	2012/13	96	94	91	90	89	
Islington	2007/8	85	89	69	42	43	27%
	2012/13	98	96	92	87	86	
Havering	2007/8	88	83	77	68	67	9%
	2012/13	96	94	91	89	87	
Brent Teaching	2007/8	91	89	76	42	43	19%
	2012/13	96	90	92	88	88	
Croydon	2007/8	91	88	77	70	61	13%
	2012/13	94	92	87	76	76	
LONDON AVERAGE	2007/8	85	84	74	50	49	18%
	2012/13	94	91	87	80	81	
Enfield	2007/8	80	72	74	50	45	14%
	2012/13	91	89	83	80	74	
Hackney	2007/8	n/a	n/a	n/a	n/a	n/a	20%
	2012/13	91	84	86	77	84	
Lewisham	2007/8	80	77	61	44	45	18%
	2012/13	90	89	86	71	71	
Kensington and Chelsea[b]	2007/8	95	93	86	n/a	n/a	22%
	2012/13	89	82	81	74	73	
Sutton and Merton[c]	2007/8	85	82	78	63	68	S = 11% M = 19%
	2012/13	89	88	81	67	69	
Westminster[d]	2007/8	81	84	n/a	n/a	n/a	24%
	2012/13	82	77	77	77	76	

15

Table 3b: Immunisation inequalities – a snapshot (continued)

Former PCTs: positioned by imms uptake 2012/13	GP–CHIS data management & IT solutions 2008-13	Index of ethnic diversity 2011: white British[e]	Relative deprivation levels[f]	Dom. visiting / Community Imms Clinics?	Average patients per GP practice 1000s[g]	Poss. levers & interventions for increased uptake including:[h]
Tower Hamlets	Fully automated system (EMIS)	31%	Very High	None	7.7	LES financial incentive for GP networks; GP Practice training on call/recall
Hillingdon	Rio; manual input; CHIS expanded with back-end 'RIO Report Manager'	52%	Low	DV & Clinics	5.9	high DV intervention / Routine data cleansing
Islington	Rio & data warehouse; Semi-automated transfer 2009-13; currently manual transfer[i]	48%	High	Clinics, including Saturdays	6	Improved data quality
Havering	Rio; Semi-automated data transfer installed during period	83%	Low	None	4.9	Circulation of GP CIP performance among practices
Brent Teaching	RiO & data warehouse (Brent Reporting Portal)	18%	Medium	Clinics; short-term DV only	4.8	Imms specialist for Somali community;
Croydon	ePEX Manual/email transfer	47%	Medium	None	6.3	Immunisation champion (temporary) 2012/13
LONDON AVERAGE		45%			5.8	
Enfield	RiO Manual/email	41%	Medium	None	5.3	Work with under-performing GP Practices
Hackney	RiO Semi-automated transfer	36%	Very High	Clinics; limited DV	6.4	Extended clinic opening for Orthodox Jewish population
Lewisham	Rio & data warehouse; Semi-automated transfer	42%	Medium to High	Clinics; Targeted MMR DV	7	Improved data collection & cleansing
Kensington and Chelsea	Rio: Manual/ email transfer	39%	Low to Medium	Weekly clinics NB reduced immunisation team	4.6	N/A: apparent reduction in uptake
Sutton and Merton	RiO Semi-automated transfer	S = 71% M = 19%	S = Low M = Low to Medium	None	7.3	Improved governance, info flows and management
Westminster	RiO + CDRIntell Vaccination and Immunisation module	35%	Medium	None NB reduced immunisation team	5	N/A: apparent reduction in uptake

Key to notes on Table 3b (previous pages)

a) Source: Communities.gov.uk. We consider these figures only approximate, due to the difficulties of capturing accurate data of population inflow and outflow. The population turnover does not include internal movement, which can also have complicating implications for immunisation.

b) Uptake may be higher than reported due to possible lack of systematic reporting of immunisation delivery by private practice.

c) Possible exclusion of data for vaccinations by 5th birthday 2012-13; coverage may be higher.

d) Uptake may be higher than reported due to possible lack of systematic reporting of immunisation delivery by private practice.

e) ONS, Census 2011.

f) Source: Trust for London and New Policy Institute, 2010. Levels are much generalised; there are for instance pockets of high deprivation in Westminster and Kensington & Chelsea.

g) London practices have on average fewer patients than the national average (6,650), but at the same time have lower than average practice staff per GP (London: 2.1; England: 2.5). Sources: The King's Fund, 2012 General Practice in London; apho.org (Public Health England) GP Practice data for 2012; accessed Oct 2013.

h) 'Possible', since outcomes have not been scientifically measured. Representatives cited improved data quality as a principal lever for increased uptake, with some emphasising the importance of aspiration and dedication (interviews or email exchanges with 2020health; Aug – Oct 2013).

i) The borough has recently experienced technical problems and has returned to manual GP-CHIS transfer.

4. The changing CIP landscape

When the NHS reorganised itself in 2013, instituting 211 CCGs (up from 152 Primary Care Trusts), it created the opportunity for a more localised response to population needs.[15] CCGs are charged with the commissioning of secondary care services, much community care and some primary care that falls outside of the General Medical Services contract. Because Childhood Immunisation is delivered by GP practices, commissioning thereof lies with NHS England, not with CCGs due to potential conflict of interest. Immunisation is therefore one of the few areas of healthcare commissioning that has become more centralised under the new system, not less.

4.1 The CIP structure, pre-reforms

Primary Care Trusts (PCTs) were 'statutory NHS bodies responsible for commissioning most health services and for improving public health'.[16] Prior to April 2013 there was a great deal of PCT-restructuring in anticipation of the wholesale move to CCGs, and accordingly some support mechanisms for the Childhood Immunisation Programme were beginning to change. However up until that time, all aspects of the Programme were highly localised, with PCTs fully in charge of CIP commissioning, support and governance.

Though it was a matter of judgement as to how PCTs should support the local CIP, it was standard to have an immunisation coordinator on the ground working alongside General Practice – encouraging staff, advising on best practice, keeping clinicians up to date on changes to policy, and compiling COVER data. Some coordinators also offered immunisation training. Coordinators would report to the immunisation lead at the PCT Board, sometimes the director of public health. Monitoring of the CIP was the role of commissioners, while provider standards (from 2008) were scrutinised by the Care Quality Commission.

As previously noted, virtually all PCTs from around 2007 worked hard to improve data quality and flow, and many invested in new Child Health Information Systems. Catch-up campaigns and the widening of access to services (e.g. domiciliary visiting, or running community immunisation clinics for unregistered 0-5s) varied from one PCT to another. Variation was due not just to perceived local needs but also to the priority level set for childhood immunisation.

From 2007 up until March 2013, nearly every PCT in England saw year on year rises in immunisation coverage. The achievements owed much to high-quality strategic planning and CIP implementation at the local level. Even though significant variation of uptake remained, many working in immunisation were – and are – justifiably proud of their hard work.

4.2 The CIP structure, post-reforms

Childhood Immunisation Programme delivery has remained GP practice-led, but CIP commissioning now lies with NHS England (formerly the NHS Commissioning Board). Public Health England, which came into full effect in April 2013, exists to protect the nation's health and address inequalities, ensuring that there are 'effective arrangements in place nationally and locally for preparing, planning and responding to health protection concerns'[17] – those of course including child immunisation. Diagram 4a presents what we have understood (at the time of reporting) to be the basic pathway overview of CIP delivery and support.

---

15. See, for example, NHS Clinical Commissioners statement, July 2013. Available: http://www.nhscc.org/wp-content/uploads/2012/06/NHSCC-response-Monitor_NHSE-How-can-NHS-payments-system-work-July-2013.pdf p.2: 'The Health and Social Care reforms have given CCGs the autonomy and space to make clinically led commissioning decisions on behalf of their local populations'.
16. NHS Confederation, 2011: The Legacy of Primary Care Trusts
17. Public Health England, April 2013: Our priorities for 2013/14.

Diagram 4a: CIP delivery and support: principal pathways (& variables)**

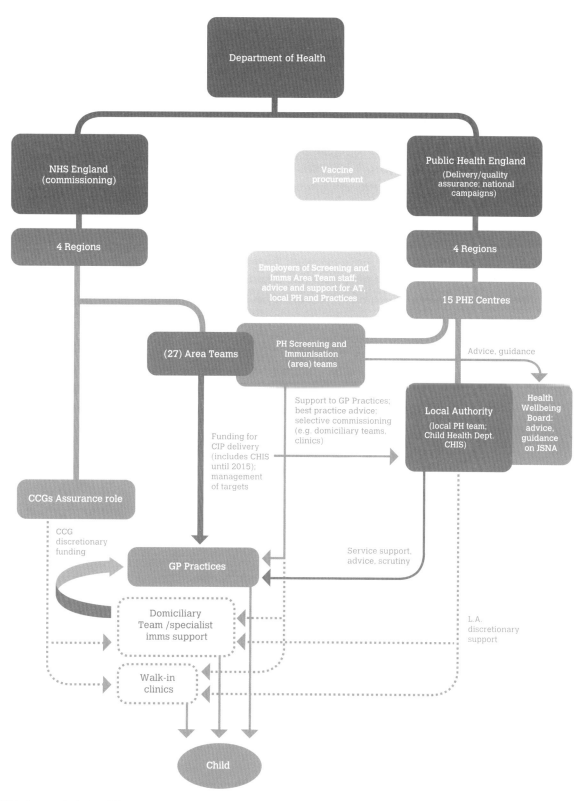

*This diagram of principal CIP delivery and support structures reflects the system as it
appeared to us at the time of reporting (November 2013), based on public-domain information
and interviews with immunisation staff at the 'area' and local level.

NHS England is divided into four commissioning regions[18] in which there sit a total of 27 Areas Teams. Each team commissions a range of primary and community healthcare services, including immunisation, for a large area that may formerly have been administered by four or five separate PCTs. In each NHS England Area Team sits a Public Health Screening and Immunisation team, whose personnel 'provide accountability and leadership for the commissioning of the [Screening and Immunisation] programmes and…provide system leadership'.[19] The Screening and Immunisation team may itself commission specific services such as domiciliary teams or community clinics;[20] otherwise they are effectively separate from the commissioning arm. Their key role is to facilitate excellence at the local General Practice level, providing service support and advice, and to ensure that high-quality immunisation training is available for providers; the team itself is not commissioned to provide training.[21] The NHS England Area Team, with support from Screening and Immunisation, hold providers to account. Many working in Screening and Immunisation teams were formerly local (PCT) immunisation coordinators, whose posts were abolished under the reforms.

Further support for the CIP is given by a Public Health team who sit within the Local Authority. Councils now have a Public Health role and are responsible for ensuring that the health needs of the local population are met. Reporting to a Health and Protection manager, PH staff supporting immunisation will be engaged in other areas of healthcare support also. Local immunisation support is therefore a coordinated effort between Local Authority Public Health and the Area Team.

Additional layers of support may be given by specialist immunisation staff – or teams, where they exist – whose role might range from providing clinical advice to delivering domiciliary immunisation and community clinics for unregistered children. They might also provide training for practice nurses. Such local additions to CIP support are typically commissioned (discretionally) by PHE Area Teams or by CCGs. Support may also be funded by a smaller NHS health body (e.g. a CPG[22]) or the Local Authority.

Diagram 4a does not show all the potential support and advice pathways at the higher organisational level.

Commissioning Support Units may have very little involvement in immunisation, as their chief relationship is with CCGs.

England's **12 Clinical Senates** may offer strategic clinical advice and leadership to CCGs, PHE and H&W Boards on a geographical basis, but the extent of their involvement in the CIP is unclear. Covering the same geographical territory as the Senates are **Strategic Clinical Networks**, which may contribute to increased pathway integration for child services, desperately needed for hard to reach children.

Health and Wellbeing Boards are cited as a potential source of strategic immunisation support at the local level, leading on the Join Strategic Needs Assessment and setting priority levels for the CIP.

Another local role is being fulfilled by **Healthwatch** (replacing Local Involvement Networks, LINks), an independent advocate for consumers of health and social care, and a statutory committee of the Care Quality Commission. Healthwatch may or may not need to engage with the CIP.

18. North of England; Midlands and East England, London (integrated region and centre); South of England
19. PHE/NHS England May 2013: Immunisation and Screening National Delivery Framework and Local Operating Model. P. 7
20. 2020health interview with Essex Area Team manager, October 2013
21. PHE/NHS England, May 2013: Immunisation & Screening National Delivery Framework & Local Operating Model: p. 24 'Developing education and training strategies – Identifying requirements for professional development in screening and ensuring that training for providers is commissioned.'
22. Clinical Programme Group

4.3 Some issues around support for the CIP

Compared with the localised PCT-driven programme, the CIP now appears more complex in terms of pathways of policy and influence, and delivery and support. Roles have changed and new organisations have come into being. Many experts we interviewed stressed that elements of the system, particularly around training and advice for practice nurses, were unclear – some key protocols do not yet exist. The sense of a lack of real 'ownership' of the system was considered problematic also, with accountability pathways difficult to define in absolute terms. This extends to the assurance role of CCGs: what is the meaning of their 'duty of quality improvement',[23] given the absence of CCG commissioning responsibilities in immunisation?

It is recognised that some Public Health posts are yet to be filled in a number of Screening and Immunisation teams.[24] And a number of localities claim to have lost immunisation support staff on the ground, beyond the decommissioning of local immunisation coordinator posts, which is creating further challenges.

Such is the context for considering learning and best practice in Sections 5 & 6: these issues and challenges of course have a significant bearing on staff confidence within England's CIP, a lack of which will almost certainly spell a reduction of uptake, in the short-term at least.

23. PHE/NHS England, May 2013. Immunisation & Screening National Delivery Framework & Local Operating Model. P. 42: 'CCGs will have a duty of quality improvement and this extends to primary medical care services delivered by GP practices such as immunisation and screening services.'
24. Information from 2020health workshop and interviews

5. National-level action and strategies

5.1 Defining roles and bringing clarity to the system

The new landscape for the Childhood Immunisation Programme, as Section 4 outlined, is perhaps little changed in terms of its ground-level delivery structures, but commissioning, support and governance systems have shifted considerably.

Whether the more centralised approach of CIP commissioning and governance will be more efficient long term is unclear. Will the system in fact become more bureaucratic with a greater number of partners involved in decision making?

Some problems have already surfaced. We were told by interviewees, repeatedly, that there is some confusion over who is responsible for funding and providing practice nurse immunisation training, and who immunisers should go to for specialist advice. We also found a lack of clarity as to how local authorities should make the case to commissioners for any new intervention. What happens if Local Government and commissioners (in Area Teams) do not agree on strategy?

Drawing upon our interviews, we turn to the most often cited issues that demand urgent attention.

5.1.1 Accountability and governance: who is ultimately responsible?

Key support and delivery roles have been identified within the CIP, but accountability, oversight and governance are much harder to define. A number of our interviewees painted a picture of a system that is not giving clear messages to its key stakeholders.

No one has contacted me, and we've had no meetings since April. Previously we'd meet every 3–6 months.

Local immunisation support

A lack of clear accountability fuels complications around the disaggregation of budgets. If commissioners claim there is no money available for a particular course of action deemed necessary by CCGs, or local Public Health and its Health & Wellbeing board, then each party may blame shift if the system fails. Though neither CCGs nor Local Authority have commissioning mandates for immunisation, they are still responsible for immunisation support, challenge and scrutiny.

We found that in certain areas key immunisation partners are not being engaged in the strategic planning of immunisation. Local NHS and Public Health staff supporting immunisation are being overlooked by commissioners and Public Health Area Teams; in one locality we heard that no official contact had been made at all, five months into the new system. This breakdown of communication begs the question as to who is responsible for ensuring that commissioners and PH Area Teams are engaging all local immunisation support staff?

The arrangements are so inordinately complicated. I can't always work out who's meant to be doing what.

Interviewee, on the new CIP landscape

There was also variation in understanding as to how local immunisation support should make their case for changes to strategy or new interventions. It was understood by some that NHS England Area Teams, with embedded support from Public

Health Screening and Immunisation Teams, have responsibility for all immunisation commissioning, including domiciliary teams and community clinics, and interventions such as mobile units. At the same time, some CCGs are choosing to fund domiciliary immunisation services, even though this is not part of their mandate.

The DH needs to recognise the substantial variation that exists across the country in CIP management and commissioning structures. It is their task to shore up stability in the CIP, something only possible by bringing greater clarity to the system.

I have asked NHS England on a couple of occasions about their plans, and I have not heard back. This is a frustration shared with other colleagues in local authorities, I think.

Interviewee, Public Health

Recommendation	Action to be taken by:
1. Identify clear pathways of accountability (not just 'roles'): locally, sub-regionally (e.g. Area Teams) and regionally.	DH
2. Identify the organisation(s) responsible for ensuring efficient information sharing and partnership working between all stakeholders.	DH
3. Make clear the role and expectations of CCGs in their 'duty of quality improvement'.	DH
4. Make clear the expectations of local Public Health where requested strategies are refused by NHS England.	DH
5. Make clear as to whether local organisations such as CCGs are expected to give financial support to immunisation services – and if so, define circumstances.	DH

5.1.2 Provider Immunisation Training

There is great confusion around the provision of immunisation training for the simple reason that the system is still in flux and few protocols actually exist. Previously the immunisation coordinator either delivered immunisation training or at least acted as sign-poster. Now, with local coordinator posts decommissioned, many practice staff do not know the identity of the training provider, nor even who to question about the delivery of training; further, not all local immunisation support staff appear to know the answer.[25]

In many cases there are not the courses available for [GP nurses] to go on…the programmes are not there to offer. NHS England could have been more proactive on this to my mind.

Public Health Nurse

---

25. Information communicated and corroborated by several interviewees

Whilst Area Teams are currently charged with ensuring that high-quality training exists, no specific body or organisation has been appointed or commissioned to deliver this. We found several different models of immunisation training delivery; for example by:

- **immunisation clinical co-ordinator**

- **consultant paediatrician**

- **Area Team member**

- **nurse immunisation specialist**

- **private provider**

In some cases, training is on offer but not officially commissioned. A few interviewees felt that local staff members were providing the service out of good will and necessity, continuing their roles from PCT days. In other localities, training was being commissioned by CCGs.

The lack of clarity in the system around such a fundamental aspect of training delivery is troubling staff at ground level. Compounding the problem, Practice managers and GPs, while responsible for ensuring employees are appropriately trained, are confused as to who should be paying for training.

Training is vital to enable primary care staff to work to Patient Group Directions: with a changing and evolving immunisation programme, the need for ensuring ready access to ongoing training becomes all the more critical.

The RCN are shortly to publish an updated training guidance document which clarifies how to commission and develop training programmes according to Health Protection Agency standards and the current curriculum. It will also include a detailed competency framework, which will be of particular value to practice managers in their role of assessing staff competence and knowledge.[26] However the document is not intended to address questions around specific commissioning structures and funding responsibilities.

Recommendation	Action to be taken by:
6. Commissioning responsibilities around immunisation training need to be clearly defined. This should include guidance to General Practice as to whether it is responsible for any funding of training.	NHS England

---

26. Competence and knowledge according to National Minimum Standards and Core Curriculum for Immunisation Training (HPA, 2005)

5.1.3 Immunisation advice

To whom should providers such as practice nurses and community nurses go for immunisation advice? Previously the obvious source was the local immunisation coordinator; if they were not able to answer the question, they would at least be able to signpost the nurse for advice. With few immunisation coordinators now in post,[27] a key component of the immunisation support chain has disappeared and not always have local GP practices been informed of new contacts for specialist advice.

Administrative problems, deriving from Public Health's move into Local Government, have compounded the problem. We heard of some cases where communication between immunisation support and General Practice broke down in part due to incomplete NHS email lists transferring over to Public Health at the Local Authority. Practices in some areas were not informed of important developments within the CIP for a number of months.

We have children with complex immunisation histories and we don't know who to go to for advice.

Interviewee, July 2013

While administrative issues are gradually being ironed out, there remains confusion within the system because pathways of immunisation advice have not been established. And advice needs to be readily available, as questions often arise while parents and children are attending clinic. Returning an answer 24 hours later represents a missed opportunity.

Every locality needs to establish for their providers a clear advice pathway, with experts identified for specific types of question. Some questions will have a local bearing, and the Local Health Protection Unit may be able to provide an answer. However only sometimes will the HPU be able to return an immediate answer to the caller, this depending on the availability of the appropriate staff member. Questions may also be fielded by local immunisation specialist nurses or consultant paediatricians. It is important that additional contact numbers are provided in the case of consultant absence or staff sickness.

Expertise among immunisation leads is patchy, and none of the support from Public Health England is well joined up.

Interviewee, Aug 2013

On a regional level, advice may be given by the Regional Paediatric Infectious Disease Unit. However it is our understanding that this does not represent a routine advice pathway for local immunisation providers.

Recommendation	Action to be taken by:
7. Each CIP provider should have access to a clear immunisation advice pathway, with contact numbers provided at the local and regional level.	Area Teams Local Public Health

---

27. Some community trusts have funded a local immunisation co-ordinator post.

Child immunisation is currently delivered within a system where expertise is unevenly scattered. There is consequently considerable need for support from a national immunisation advice line, or information hub, accessible online. A model for this may be VACCSline, established by the Oxford Vaccine Group. It is currently a regional organisation and has limited online capability. But creating a national role for an organisation like VACCSline would bring enormous benefit to the CIP, particularly where specialist advice and support are needed by more isolated immunisation providers.

Recommendation	Action to be taken by:
8. Expert advice needs to be readily accessible to immunisers in both urban and remote regions. A national immunisation advice line, staffed by experts and with wide online functionality, would be a highly valued resource.	DH

5.1.4 Conclusion: the impact of uncertainty

New systems take time to settle down and embed. It is not surprising that elements within the immunisation landscape remain unclear. But the confusion surrounding training and advice threatens to undermine recent success within the CIP. Specifically, it endangers some of the core values of best practice as identified in Joint Strategic Needs Assessment (JSNA) guidelines,[28] which recommend that immunisers:

1. Keep up to date with changes to policy and parental concerns
2. Ensure they have access to current vaccine policy
3. Ensure they know who to contact when they need further advice or information
4. Attend regular training updates
5. Make time to discuss parental concerns about immunisation
6. Be knowledgeable and confident
7. Promote vaccination

Many of these best practice standards (arguably all except 2 & 5) are under threat by current system confusion. If General Practice immunisers are confused and feel unsupported within the system, Public Health should not expect to see stability in the CIP. Indeed a number of experts we interviewed expect to see a downturn in immunisation coverage. It is up to the DH and Public Health England to anticipate this problem and fast-track appropriate action.

28. Good Practice Template for the Immunisation Component of the Joint Strategic Needs Assessment. 2012

5.2 Health visitors:
accessing the hard-to-reach

While the service infrastructure of the Childhood Immunisation Programme is usually very good for stable families, it often breaks down for hard-to-reach groups, particularly those in temporary accommodation, children in care, and traveller communities. Solutions are needed both at the national and local level to respond to this problem. Here we discuss the role of Health Visitors, while in Section 6.1 we consider more generally the widening of access to immunisation services.

5.2.1 The Healthy Child Programme

Health Visitors have a vital role to play in the Healthy Child Programme (HCP), an early intervention and prevention public health programme introduced in 2009[29] involving screening, immunisation, health and development reviews for children (0-5s) and parenting support. To strengthen the HCP the DH pledged to increase the number of health visitors by 4,200 (approximately 40% rise)[30] between 2011 and 2015.[31] While the DH sets mandates and develops health visiting policy, NHS England, through its 27 Area Teams, is responsible for commissioning health visitors – a task that will pass to local authorities in 2015.

In their national priorities for local delivery, the DH states that the HCP will 'support the delivery of…an increase in the proportion of children who complete immunisation by recommended ages.'[32] While not formally tasked with delivering immunisation, the health visitor team works with general practice to ensure that families have access to the services of the HCP, which should be 'made available in convenient local settings', including Sure Start Children's Centres, health centres and family homes.[33]

Health visitors are trained nurses or midwives who hold post-graduate specialist practitioner qualifications. Working in the field of child and family health and wellbeing, they lead and deliver The Healthy Child Programme (extending from pregnancy through to 5 years). The health visitor's role within the Childhood Immunisation Programme includes:

- Promotion of immunisation to parents

- Referring of unregistered or defaulting children on to (or back to) GPs

- Checking the child's immunisation record (in Redbook) when home visiting

- Assessing children's immunisation status at Sure Start centres, nurseries and other pre-school organisations

- Updating immunisation data on the Child Health Information System and feeding through information for the GPs' system

- Meeting regularly with GPs to update them on which new-born children in the area have not been immunised

Some ambiguity may be read in the mandate given to health visitors: on the one hand there is no explicit remit for health visitors to provide immunisation; on the other, they have to work to ensure access to all elements of the HCP for registered and unregistered children, and support timely immunisation.

---

29. The design of the HCP incorporates the (previous) Child Health Surveillance programme
30. There were around 10,000 health visitors in England as of September 2010. Source: Department of Health, 2010. Equality Analysis: Health Visiting Programme.
31. Department of Health: Health Visitor Implementation Plan, 2011-15.
32. Department of Health, 2009. Healthy Child Programme
33. DH 2012 Health Visitor factsheet

Very few health visitors immunise these days. With the CIP delivered primarily (sometimes exclusively) from GP practices, roles have shifted. Moreover, health visitors already manage wide caseloads and child safeguarding and protection have increased; few want to take on more responsibilities. It also of course needs to be recognised that GPs are paid to deliver immunisation; health visitors are not. At the same time, the health visitor team is the one of the very few burgeoning resources within healthcare. With CIP support in short supply in many localities, is now the time for health visitors to take an active role in delivering opportunistic immunisation?

5.2.2 Health visitors and immunisation

At this current time, where domiciliary services and community clinics do not exist for CIP support, health visitors typically refer defaulters or unregistered children back or on to GPs. However there is no guarantee that parents will attend clinic. A parent might be disorganised and forget, or feel too busy to attend; they might be ambivalent about immunisation and regard it as low priority, or have difficulty mobilising a large family to clinic. Some, due to language barriers or illiteracy, will have difficulty understanding appointment times, while others may be vaccine-resistant.

The arguments for involving health visitors in immunisation delivery have much to do with issues of equity – not just in terms of access, but also where the health interests of the child are potentially subjugated by a parent's busy schedule or lack of concern. It is essential that health visitors work diligently to refer children on to GPs – not just for immunisation – and this should be a targeted outcome. But often risks are being taken, those of missed immunisations, which could be mitigated if members of the health visitor team have the ability and inclination to vaccinate.

Student health visitors often want to learn how to vaccinate and don't understand why they can't.

Comment from immunisation workshop, September 2013

The historic arguments against health visitors vaccinating – those of heavy workloads and increased safeguarding – carry less weight if health visiting teams are expanding in capacity. Health visitors are well placed to give domiciliary immunisation, if only as a last resort in the absence of a specialised domiciliary immunisation team. The service would present particular value for disabled parents, for looked-after children and for families who are routinely disengaged with the CIP. Traveller communities, whose members are often reluctant to register with a GP, could also benefit from this service where it is coordinated by a Local Authority traveller representative.

It was the perception of a number of experts at our workshop that student health visitors are generally keen to take on immunisation training. We recommend that immunisation, as part of the Healthy Child Programme, forms part of the routine training for health visitors to make opportunity for widened access, even if immunisation delivery itself is not mandated for all health visitors on the ground.[34]

Recommendation	Action to be taken by:
9. Immunisation, as part of the Healthy Child Programme, should be a mandatory component of health visitor training so to maximise opportunities for access to services. HV delivery of immunisation should only occur where parents are considered unlikely to attend GP settings or child health clinics – thus as a last resort.	DH

34. If a health visitor (student or fully qualified) is a registered nurse and has undergone immunisation foundation training (meeting Public Health England and local mandatory training criteria), they can already work to Patient Group Directions in the delivery of immunisation.

5.3 Directed Enhanced Service (DES) payments: a time for change?

5.3.1 The DES

GP practices do not have to provide child immunisation, although the vast majority do, receiving payment under the 'Additional Service' contract. If a practice achieves an average 70% uptake for the five-in-one vaccine (DTaP/IPV/Hib), MMR and MenC, they qualify for a Directed Enhanced Service payment. If the practice achieves 90% uptake, they receive a payment three times greater. These payments are directly related to the number of children they immunise.[35]

5.3.2 What are the concerns?

While targets and incentives are embedded in the NHS system, there is an important question to ask as to whether the targets for any current year should necessarily be the same as the targets set previously. The DES 70% and 90% thresholds may have been deemed appropriate and useful at one time when uptake around England was generally poor; but these thresholds are now severely criticised by many working in immunisation, principally because they do not reflect the recommended 95% target set by the World Health Organisation as critical to herd immunity.

Many are asking why it is that GPs are being financially rewarded for hitting sub-optimal targets. Particularly, why reward GPs for 70% uptake when that figure represents system failure? Moreover, according to many we interviewed, it appears that the DES does not incentivise optimal uptake because once a practice achieves 90%, and receives payment, there is no incentive to raise uptake further. Increasing uptake to 95% may require significantly more work for little financial reward.

The GP tariff bears no relation to what we actually need to achieve in terms of herd immunity

Interviewee, Public Health immunisation support

A second DES frustration raised by experts we interviewed concerns the actual reporting of immunisation by GP practices. Practices are required to report immunisations in a timely fashion to the Child Health Department, where data are loaded onto the Child Health Information System (CHIS). This is the information that creates COVER statistics for immunisation uptake in the locality. However, the DES is not linked to these data, but rather to data sent to the EXETER system. GP practices have a financial interest in feeding accurate information through to EXETER, but not the CHIS. Further, whereas timely immunisation is vital to COVER data, DES payments may be made even where the Practice fails to immunise according to the 24- or 60-month COVER schedule; a vaccination given several months late for COVER, will still qualify under EXETER for a DES payment.

In two essential contexts, the DES is misaligned to the targets set by both the World Health Organisation and England's Department of Health.

---

35. NHS England: General Medical Services Statement of Financial Entitlements Directions 2013.

5.3.3 How should the DES be changed?

Though the DES problem was raised both in interviews and at the workshop, those critical of the system (in fact the majority of interviewees) did not all offer suggestions on precise terms and conditions of change, but rather said that there needed to be alignment with WHO and DH objectives for vaccination uptake.

Most interviewees who expressed an opinion recommended a 95% threshold for the top DES payment, but none appeared to have firm ideas as to the appropriate lower threshold rise. One thought a 70% to 80% rise to be a step in the right direction.

A key question for policy makers is, will raising the DES thresholds, for example to 80% and 95%, create a disincentive among some practices to attain higher uptake if they are already struggling to reach 70% or 90%? However this same argument will have applied to 70% and 90% thresholds previously, at a time when uptake was generally much lower and practices routinely struggled to achieve 90%. Now, with better data systems, improved learning and greater public awareness, 90% uptake in most areas of England is expected. Even in London, as table 3b shows, average uptake for the primary 5-in-1 and MenC vaccinations is above 90%. Recent figures for MMR uptake in England, thanks to the 2013 catch-up campaign, stands at 92.3 at 24 months.[36] This is the crux as to why many believe it is now time to reconfigure the thresholds.

> *We need to incentivise GP practices to hit 95% and the DES is not helping*
>
> **Interviewee, immunisation specialist**

5.3.4 Would three DES thresholds be better than two?

Three thresholds may sound like more bureaucracy, but it is in effect what some localities have implemented with a Local Enhanced Service (LES) 95% uptake reward, on top of the DES 90% payment, with the payment itself coming from (what was at the time) the PCT. Tower Hamlets have pursued this strategy on a GP-network basis and consider it highly effective. In their case, GP practices are clustered into networks with an appointed manager and coordinator; each practice within the network has to achieve 95% uptake for all network members to secure payment.[37] [38]

Local authorities may want to consider this LES GP network-rewarding strategy, although other strategic needs may have greater priority. But if something similar was instituted as national policy, then a 95% payment could be funded through a reconfiguration of existing DES payments: the thresholds and ratio of payments perhaps (80%) 1: (90%) 2.5: (95%) 3.5.

---

36. http://www.nursingtimes.net/nursing-practice/clinical-zones/immunology/mmr-uptake-at-its-highest-levels/5063740.article
37. 2020health interviews: 19 July / 16 September 2013
38. Tower Hamlets Joint Strategic Needs Assessment 2010–11

5.3.5 Timely reporting

In terms of encouraging timely reporting from GPs, opinion was again consistent only on the matter of a revision of the process itself. All criticised the system's procedure to allow rewards for GP Practices who deliver late immunisation, and some thought that DES payments should be linked to CHIS/COVER data.

Aligning with COVER?

Bringing the DES payments into alignment with COVER data again raises problems for some practices, who may struggle with a population that has immunisation as low priority and do not always attend clinic at designated times.[39] The extra time period, allowed by the DES, gives opportunity for catch-up, even if these children do not receive such timely immunisation.

But to remain with the status quo is to uphold a system that is clearly fighting with itself: it is difficult to make a solid case as to why such conflicting agendas of Public Health and GPs should be in the public interest.

Investment in data flow over the last few years has increased capability for timely immunisation and reporting: if there ever was a robust argument for not aligning the DES with COVER data, it is a much less convincing argument now. This is a high level debate that urgently needs to happen.

Recommendation	Action to be taken by:
10. (General) DES payment thresholds are widely considered unfit for purpose and obstacles to increased uptake. Now is the time – following the reforms – to review strategy and raise thresholds.	DH, in consultation with: NHS England PHE
11. (Specific) The lowest DES threshold should be raised from 70% to 80%. We also recommend a three-tier DES system that incentivises optimal uptake, with a new 95% reward facilitated through a reduction of the 90% payment; the relative scale of financial reward thus rising: 1 (80%): 2.5 (90%): 3.5 (95%).	DH, in consultation with: NHS England PHE
12. Public health and GP Practice need to be focused on the same targets: DES payments should therefore be aligned to COVER, with the Child Health Information System used as the source of data to calculate GP payments. This is critical to encouraging General Practice in timely immunisation and reporting.	DH

---

39. The parent's perception of 'low priority' may of course be influenced by access difficulties beyond their control.

5.4 Locating the data: the Summary Care Record

Immunisation information is often spread across multiple locations and may be variously found in a Child's Redbook, travel documents, a hospital unit, a GP system (NHS or private) or CHIS. Given the increased mobility of populations, there is urgent need to create a system whereby accurate records of immunisation and other important health information can be centrally located.

The most obvious available solution is the Summary Care Record – a very basic, emergency care electronic health record that typically contains essential information about the holder's ongoing medication, allergies and history of adverse reactions to medicines. This record has the potential to hold immunisation information also. As the SCR was developed as an opt-out system (rather than active opt-in), most people, whether conscious of the fact or not, have an SCR, including children.[40] Over 30 million SCRs have been created, as of September 2013, with reported opt-out standing at 1.4%.[41]

Currently used primarily for out-of-hours and emergency situations, the SCR holds considerable potential for the CIP. Indeed, considering the capability of the SCR, it is surprising that it has not already been promoted as a means to record immunisation history. The SCR can be updated and accessed from any locality by a clinical professional, as long as permission has been granted by the holder or representative.[42]

The argument for the SCR was made during our workshop, and it was acknowledged that work is underway to investigate how the Summary Care Record can be expanded and immunisations included. In theory, immunisation history can already be added to the SCR by a doctor, as long as explicit consent has been given by the patient. But immunisation status has yet to become embedded as 'core data'.[43]

In time it would be valuable to see downloadable SCRs, so individuals themselves can store and carry their own immunisation data. This would be a positive step towards the widespread use of electronic Personal Health Records (PHR). The PHR supports personal healthcare management and responsibility, and provides clinicians with comprehensive health data accessible from any location, with patient consent.

Recommendation	Action to be taken by:
13. Since most children born in England have a Summary Care Record created at birth, the electronic SCR should be promoted from the outset as a record for CIP activity, with immunisation status included as SCR 'core data'.	DH

40. http://www.nhscarerecords.nhs.uk/havescr
41. http://systems.hscic.gov.uk/scr/staff/aboutscr/benefits/scrkey
42. In emergency cases where the holder lacks capacity or is unconscious, access can be gained without holder consent.
43. Clinical Use of the Summary Care Record, 2011: available http://systems.hscic.gov.uk/scr/staff/clinusejul.pdf

6. Local-level action and strategies

6.1 Widening access to immunisation: home visiting and community clinics

....

Commissioners…should improve access to immunisation services for those with transport, language or communication difficulties, and those with physical or learning disabilities. For example, provide longer appointment times, walk-in vaccination clinics, services offering extended hours and mobile or outreach services.

National Institute for Health and Clinical Excellence[44]

....

General Practice is the key commissioned provider of the childhood immunisation programme, but practices themselves have limited resources to pursue parents who default, refuse, or simply do not respond at all. Previously, PCTs in many localities commissioned home visiting teams and/or community walk-in clinics to improve uptake, but this was by no means a universal strategy. Reviewing activity from 2008 to March 2013, some PCTs, such as Walsall in the West Midlands, South Tyneside and the London borough of Tower Hamlets, managed high uptake without. Others, such as Salford and the London borough of Hillingdon, have seen domiciliary services as essential to increased uptake; while Kensington & Chelsea chose to decommission its domiciliary service in 2011/12 but retain community immunisation clinics.

In April 2013 the responsibility for investment in immunisation services transferred from PCTs to NHS England, with the deployment of funds through 27 Area Teams and associated Public Health Screening and Immunisation teams. The case for community immunisation clinics and domiciliary services needs to be now (re-)reviewed for each locality under the new commissioning arrangements, with the participation of local authorities, CCGs and Health and Wellbeing Boards. If some PCTs previously chose not to commission widened access, the question now is should NHS England continue with that same strategy, bearing in mind NICE best practice, as quoted above?

6.1.1 Home visiting

At this current time, and with no mandate for health visitors to be delivering home immunisation (See Section 5.2), many localities have no domiciliary immunisation provision. Judging from comments made at the workshop, there is mixed opinion among professionals about the need for such a service, or where it works best.

On the subject of the measles vaccine, NICE's report Reducing differences in the uptake of immunisations (2009)[45] makes the claim:

Economic modelling showed that at current levels of immunisation [2009]… home visits (likely to be the most expensive means of increasing coverage by one percentage point) would be a cost effective use of NHS resources. The implication is that almost any method of increasing coverage would be cost effective.

....

44. NICE website: Providing information on, and access to, immunisation services. Accessed 15.10.13. Available: http://tinyurl.com/pjz838j
45. Report available: http://www.nice.org.uk/nicemedia/live/12247/45497/45497.pdf

NICE asserts home visiting cost-efficiency for 'both high and low immunisation coverage'. Of course, uptake has much improved since 2009, so an updated statement by NICE, working from current COVER statistics, is very much needed for clarity around best practice.

Some localities, such as Hillingdon in London, Dudley in the West Midlands, and West Sussex, have sustained or deployed new domiciliary immunisation to target defaulters or the hard to reach; but it was the perception, if not experience, of some we interviewed that a significant number of domiciliary teams have been disbanded with the reforms.[46]

If this means that traditional domiciliary teams are considered only occasionally cost-effective, then other domiciliary models surely need to be considered. For example, where uptake is already reasonably high, a cost-efficient domiciliary model may involve a small dedicated team delivering immunisation across multiple localities. With NHS England commissioning through its Area Teams, this becomes a much more viable option than previously, where coordinated commissioning would have been required among several PCTs.

Some kind of domiciliary immunisation service, whether specific to a locality or working across multiple localities, appears to be a necessary strategy for accessing various 'hard to reach' groups (see Hillingdon inset). While it is perhaps not desirable to create dependency on such a service, domiciliary visiting may well be the only realistic option for a significant proportion of unregistered children or routine defaulters. Commissioners and Public Health strategists need to consider not so much whether a person can attend clinic, but whether they will.

6.1.2 Community clinics

Community immunisation clinics, where they exist, are normally held at children's centres, but could also be delivered at Sure Start centres, nurseries and other pre-school activity locations. Health visitors, working with childcare or education staff and parents, are tasked with checking the immunisation record (including the personal child health record) of each child aged up to 5 years, whether in the home or 'when the child joins a day nursery, nursery school, playgroup, Sure Start children's centre or when they start primary school'.[47]

The health visitor should always try and refer immunisation defaulters and unregistered children on to a local GP, and indeed not all community-based immunisation services are currently made available to under-5s. Ideally, however, community immunisation clinics should be facilitating widened access for the CIP, for example in cases where:

- local GP practices opt out of giving vaccinations

- local GP practices restrict clinics to office hours, weekdays

- large families avoid GP clinics due to practice size
  (or lack of facilities to accommodate and entertain children)

- access to GP practice is less convenient

46. 2020health: comments from interviewees, August – October 2013.
47. NICE, 2009. Reducing differences in the uptake of immunisations

6. Local-level action and strategies

Saturday clinics are often made available at children's centres; in the London borough of Hackney there are even Sunday clinics for the Orthodox Jewish population.

If our workshop and interviews suggest that opinion around domiciliary immunisation services is split, there appears to be more agreement around community immunisation clinics. However, not all localities appear to have the staff to run immunisation clinics. We have already discussed the possibility of engaging suitably-trained health visitors in the task of immunisation support (Section 5.2), and otherwise NHS England will need to consider recruiting/training other community nurses for the task.

Alternatively, if Area Teams deploy area-wide mobile services (see above), the same staff could also run community immunisation clinics, restricted to specific days at different children's centres where there is not local staff capacity to implement this.

6.1.3 Can higher uptake be achieved without domiciliary services or clinics?

The London borough of Tower Hamlets, as Table 3b confirms, has high levels of population turnover, significant ethnic diversity, extensive pockets of deprivation, and an above-average number of patients per GP practice; and yet the borough, without domiciliary services or community clinics, has achieved the highest uptake in London across the full range of vaccinations under the CIP. However, their strategy for increasing uptake has relied significantly on full GP-CHIS system interoperability, together with the introduction of financial incentives (via a Local Enhanced Service – LES) for networks of GP practices to hit 95% targets (see also Section 5.3.4). The LES was supported by additional IT training for practices on the call and recall programme, and the strategy itself encouraged the sharing of learning among GP practices. Tower Hamlets also claims strong leadership and aspiration as key levers.[48] Other localities need to examine learning from Tower Hamlets and decide whether their strategic plan is in part or wholly transferable.

Recommendation	Action to be taken by:
14. The Tower Hamlets model of CIP delivery needs to be studied by all localities (where uptake remains poor) to guide JSNA priorities. This includes consideration of LES payments for GP networks where immunisation uptake reaches 95% across all practices.	Local Authorities

It is possible that some localities will consider the Tower Hamlets strategy too expensive if uptake is already high without it; some might consider it inappropriate, given the challenges around uptake specific to their area. But where uptake is low, and no domiciliary services or clinics exist, there must be urgent review as to whether the current strategy is the right one. And even where GP-CHIS systems are semi- or fully interoperable and uptake is high, there may still be good cause to introduce new services to widen access, in order to reduce inequalities and raise uptake in all areas of the locality to herd immunity levels. Just because a locality can claim a 95% uptake average, this does not necessarily represent 95% uptake in each and every district.

48. 2020health interviews: July/September 2013

Recommendation	Action to be taken by:
15. An 'Area Immunisation Task Force' should be considered for each Area to deliver mobile immunisation services to the 'hard-to-reach', as well as run community immunisation clinics in localities that lack capacity for such services.	NHS England Public Health Screening and Immunisation Area Teams

6.2 Immunisation information management

It was the considered opinion of all immunisation experts we interviewed that greater efficiency of data transfer, collection, cleansing and gleaning has been at the heart of increased uptake in many localities across England. Improved information management should be a priority activity for all local authorities: knowing the demographics and immunisation status of your population is critical.

From around 2007 there was increased activity across England to raise standards of data management. For many PCTs at that time, data flow was largely manual, with immunisation records posted or faxed from GP surgeries to the local Child Health Department, where the Child Health Information System (CHIS) would be manually updated. Immunisation information exchange from one PCT's CHIS to another was also often also by post.[49]

6.2.1 Data quality: what it means and how to achieve it

The challenge was, and still is, to bring greater electronic interoperability to immunisation data management – a challenge because CHIS and GP systems are rarely compatible. Before exploring this problem it is worth recognising what 'accurate immunisation data' actually means for both providers and Child Health Departments.

---

49. Healthcare for London: The London childhood immunisation project, Interim Report, June 2009

Table 6.2a: The value of accurate immunisation data:

1. Enables providers to see exactly when children are due for immunisation and issue reminders prior to appointment

2. Affords opportunity for efficient recall (usually by General Practice) when appointments are missed

3. Ensures against duplicate immunisations (saving NHS money, as well giving parents peace of mind)

4. Delivers meaningful COVER statistics, demonstrating to stakeholders and the general public the effectiveness of the CIP – nationally, regionally and locally

5. Brings clarity to population needs, informing decision making around access to services and catch-up strategies

6. Interprets General Practice delivery; EXETER system guides the appropriate Directed Enhanced Service payment, where applicable

Childhood Immunisation Programme data accuracy relies on four principal information flows:

• From GP practices to the Child Health Department, where information is loaded into the Child Health Information System (CHIS)

• From other immunisation providers (Children's centres, domiciliary teams, school nurses, hospitals, private clinics), some of whom will be able to update CHIS directly

• From health visitors and other community workers who are able to report on the immunisation status of unregistered or hard-to-reach children

• Out-of-Area Child Information Systems (OOA CHIS), supplying information about children moving into an area

6.2.2 Data flow

Principal child immunisation data flows

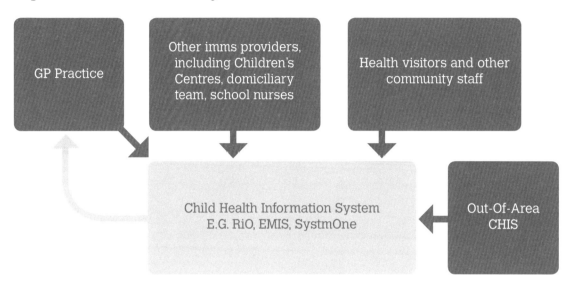

General Practice is the core centre of CIP activity – few practices opt out of administering child vaccinations. Data need to be registered on the practice system immediately after vaccination. Vaccination data should then be submitted weekly, otherwise fortnightly, to the Child Health Department. Some automated data collection systems collect immunisation data from a practice once per month. These data can then be validated and entered automatically into the CHIS within a few hours.

CIP delivery may be exclusive to GP practices in a given area, but otherwise it is common for a small proportion of child immunisation to be given by domiciliary teams or school nurses, or at Children's Centres by community staff nurses on the Health Visiting team. Health visitors rarely immunise (these days), but they are typically well-placed to find out the immunisation status of unregistered children. Once information is uploaded on the CHIS, data should then feed back to the relevant GP practices on a weekly or fortnightly basis, so practice systems can be updated.[50]

Not only does data reporting need to be timely and accurate, but the CHIS requires routine data cleansing. Best practice around data collection and cleansing has been published in the report Child Health Immunisation System: Database Cleansing (2009),[51] which provides advice on how to optimise the CHIS to accurately account for the local population and their immunisation status.

Recommendation	Action to be taken by:
16. NHS England (currently responsible for commissioning CHIS systems) needs to review its provision for routine CHIS data cleansing and gleaning, and recognise this as a priority for all Child Health Departments. This vital procedure is not yet embedded across England.	NHS England

50. Childhood Immunisation for London, August 2010. Available: http://www.londonhp.nhs.uk/wp-content/uploads/2011/03/Childhood-Immunisation-for-London-Part-B-Immunisation-Guidance.pdf
51. Available: http://www.londonhp.nhs.uk/wp-content/uploads/2011/03/Immunisation-database-cleansing-guide.pdf

6.2.3 Data challenges: system interoperability

IT solutions to data management are currently a local and national concern. Prior to 2013, Child Health Information Systems were commissioned by PCTs. From 2013 to 2015 NHS England 'will undertake responsibility for ensuring CHIS are commissioned effectively.' It will do this through its 27 Area Teams. Thereafter, responsibility for children's public health services for 0-5 year olds is expected to transfer to local authorities.[52]

The challenge for local authorities, and currently NHS England, is that CHIS and GP practice systems are rarely interoperable – most do not 'talk' to each other. Further, GP practices in a locality may be themselves using different systems (EMIS, SystmOne, Vision, etc). Work has been undertaken to at least bring greater consistency to the immunisation report format supplied by GP practices, as multiple formats have been in use.

Data flow broadly follows one or more of the following methods:

1. Manual transfer, with paper records posted or faxed from GP surgeries to the Child Health Department, where data is entered onto CHIS

2. Email transfer, with GP surgeries emailing immunisation records to the Child Health Department, where data is entered manually onto CHIS

3. Semi-automated transfer, where the GP practice extracts data with third party software and sends aggregated information via email to an agency (such as BT),[53] which then facilitates automatic entry of immunisation data onto the CHIS (e.g. RiO)

4. Automated transfer, where CHIS is fully compatible and interconnected with GP systems (using the same platform) and can extract relevant information, as programmed

Naturally, the first method is most labour intensive and open to human error, while the fourth method is least labour intensive and (in theory) the most accurate.

Only one locality we contacted – Tower Hamlets – is currently running a fully automated electronic system, since both GP practices and the Child Health Department are using EMIS. In other areas there may be part interoperability, as in Essex, where the CHIS and many GP practices are using SystmOne.

The IT situation for much of London is quite different. Nearly all London boroughs use RiO for their CHIS, which while possessing various strengths, has little compatibility with many GP systems. Another restriction of RiO is that it operates as a transactional system – it is very limited as an analytical system. Some localities (such as Hillingdon) are using back-end software on RiO to generate wider analyses and reports, whereas others have employed semi-automated 'data warehouse' solutions.

52. Department of Health, April 2013. Public Health Functions to be exercised by NHS England. CHIS Available: https://www.gov.uk/government/uploads/system/uploads/attachment_data/file/192979/28_CHIS_service_specification_VARIATION_130422.pdf
53. The agency collects Quality and Outcomes Framework data which is not patient-identifiable.

London boroughs using data warehouses include Brent, Islington, Lewisham and Westminster. The data warehouse is independent of the CHIS and GP systems. Information is received from GP practices and the CHIS, as well as from the schools census and the Demographic Batch Service. GP data may arrive in the form of an attachment to an email: the attachment has to be manually copied to an application within the data warehouse system for the data to be extracted by the programme. CHIS data flow can be fully automated and timed for overnight transfer.

Data warehouse systems can produce detailed analyses of CIP delivery – e.g. practice by practice, or domiciliary team activity – displayed in the form of tables, bar charts or pie charts as preferred. They bring greater accuracy to real-time progress on uptake and can also facilitate efficient data cleansing processes, creating cleansing logs to reduce risk of human error.

While data warehouses do not actually create CHIS and GP system interoperability, they may well be the cheapest, most secure and efficient way for NHS England and local Public Health to improve data quality and flow. Learning and best practice around data warehouses is being generated currently, but this needs wider dissemination.

Recommendation	Action to be taken by:
17. NHS England needs to improve CHIS-GP system data flow and analyses by commissioning 'third party' solutions, such as semi-automated data warehouse systems. Such systems significantly improve data quality, allow for detailed analysis of CIP delivery, and optimise call/recall activity.	NHS England

6.3 Immunisation strategies for further consideration

Here we highlight strategies that to our mind deserve further consideration and promotion as levers for increased uptake. This is not to deny a variety of other important approaches, such as opportunistic vaccination at hospitals, or London's recent 'Celebrate and Protect' project,[54] an evaluation of which was planned for autumn 2013 but not published at the time of reporting.

6.3.1 Catch up, done cheaply

Off-site catch-up immunisation strategies are sometimes undertaken with mobile units, such as Hackney's Spotty Bus campaign of 2007, which targeted schools and nurseries to deliver opportunistic vaccinations to more than 800 children.[55] Some mobile interventions have been undertaken with private nurses, due to a lack of local NHS immunisation staff, and associated costs have naturally been higher.

What is probably one of the most cost-efficient catch-up strategies of the last few years was undertaken in the borough of Halton in the North West, in 2008, which included immunisation clinics held at venues in a local shopping centre.[56]

54. A partnership between local authorities, Sanofi Pasteur MSD and the NHS. Information available from: www.spmsd.co.uk/doc.asp?catid=481&docid=912

55. Sources: http://ecdc.europa.eu/en/press/events/Documents/UK-Country-initiatives-aimed-at-improving-vaccination-uptake.pdf; also Hackney Scrutiny Commission, April 2008; Available: http://tinyurl.com/o2xejbu

56. A full account of the initiative has been published by Landes Bioscience; available (by purchase): https://www.landesbioscience.com/journals/vaccines/article/24695/

The shopping centre venues were risk-assessed by the immunisation team, infection control and the ambulance service. Four catch-up sessions (including two held at community clinics) were promoted with information postcards distributed from local shops selling school uniform (the postcard put in the bag with purchase) and the local library (the postcard put in borrowed children's books). Cards and posters were also displayed by hair salons, supermarkets, and at customer service desks in the shopping centre.

Each session was led by the immunisation coordinator and planned in collaboration with the Health Visiting Lead, and Lead Immunisation Trainer. The Health Visiting Service delivered all clinical sessions with four immunisers on site. Toys were provided in a play area and further fun and distraction was provided by a children's entertainer for part of each day.

With the locality-wide awareness initiative launched, a total of 1,025 children, identified as behind in their vaccination schedule, were invited to the catch-up sessions. It was anticipated that a minimum of 60 children per day would attend over an eight hour period, though they had staff capacity to handle much more. In fact, this two-pronged strategy resulted in nearly 100 children in attendance at each clinic – 398 in total, representing a positive response rate of 39%.

Children registered with 12 different GP practices in the PCT attended the clinics, with the majority activity taking place between 11am and 3pm. A total of 728 vaccines were administered:

- 339 MMR

- 255 pre-school booster

- 53 Hib/MenC

- 81 PCV

Halton 2008 catch-up summary:

- Four clinics, two held at a local shopping centre

- catch-up immunisations publicised locally with postcards and posters via shops and library

- targeted invites sent to 1,025 children 39% response rate, with 398 children immunised

- Toys and children's entertainer to keep waiting (and accompanying) children occupied

- Cooperation between NHS and Local Authority; maximisation of resources to keep costs to a minimum

This represents significant success. During our interviews we heard of a mobile immunisation strategy that secured a 10% response, and this was itself considered successful.

A pilot clinic previously deployed by the same Halton team (again in the shopping centre) achieved a 24% response without local promotion through the postcard/poster strategy.[57]

In terms of financial efficiency, it is recorded that the pilot session, whose delivery model informed the four subsequent catch-up clinics, came in at approximately £650; costs were kept to a minimum because the venue was provided for free by the Local Authority and the immunisation team was working within contracted hours. Screens, desks, chairs and children's toys were brought in from elsewhere.

57. The pilot was specifically MMR, so uptake may be expected to be somewhat less than a programme offering a range of vaccinations due to the legacy of the 1998 MMR scare.

Children who did not attend the catch-up clinics were referred back to their GP; it is not known how many children were subsequently immunised as a result. And what of course cannot be known is how many children attending the catch-up clinics may have otherwise (eventually) attended recall for immunisation at their local GP practice. But PCT uptake figures prior and subsequent to the catch-up campaign are compelling, with notable increased uptake for MMR1 at 24 months, identified by a 9% rise between Q4 2007 and Q3 2008.

While it is a fact that some localities with depleted immunisation teams would not be able to deploy the same strategy without 'outside' (perhaps private provider) assistance, the Halton project demonstrates how to raise awareness around the childhood immunisation programme and increase access by maximising the resources at the disposal of the NHS and Local Authority. It represents partnership working, creativity and ambition, qualities never more needed by our financially-challenged healthcare system.

Recommendation	Action to be taken by:
18. The improved dissemination of learning from successful, cost-effective catch-up strategies is much needed. Very few have been written up with robust data and published in the public domain.	LA Public Health DH

6.3.2 Targeted advertising via transport networks

It is rare to see immunisation awareness on high-profile advertising platforms these days. Whilst catch-up campaigns, such as that of MMR recently, may receive some public promotion through printed media, there appears to be little presence of immunisation as 'prevention' in either national or regional advertising.

National advertising campaigns are typically very expensive and unsustainable. However regional advertising is much cheaper and can facilitate targeted messages to at-risk populations. Regional and sub-regional advertising could be better exploited in areas such as London and Birmingham to raise awareness around childhood immunisation, and particularly the pre-school 4-in-1 booster and MMR second dose as part of an annual 'fit-for-school' strategy.

Councils often benefit from reduced advertising rates, and this is certainly the case in London. Transport advertising, including static poster advertising (at train/tube stations and bus stops), mobile advertising (on tube or bus panels) and interior screen advertising (some buses) is an approach that allows communication inter-regionally to specific districts and boroughs – even down to a specific bus stop. Bus shelter adverts outside zone one in London start at around £330 each for a fortnight (e.g. in Newham); within zone one the prices are higher, rising to as much as £3,000 in central locations such as Oxford Street. Bus (mobile) advertising is organised by bus depot rather than exact routes, so advertising becomes borough-wide rather than district-specific. Side panel advertising starts at around £320 for a two week period, per bus.[58]

58. 2020health communication with Clear Channel and CBS Outdoor. Prices correct at the time of reporting, relevant to councils, although further discounts may be available for such public health concerns.

Recommendation	Action to be taken by:
19. District-level, if not borough-wide, 'fit-for-school' immunisation advertising campaigns should be considered for local strategy, maximising transport-network and shop-window opportunities to warn at-risk populations of the dangers of missed vaccinations. It should be recognised that local Public Health is often eligible for discounted advertising rates.	LA Public Health CCGs

The same print advertisements used on transport networks can of course be distributed to GP surgeries, pharmacies and community centres for wider community circulation. Again, specific boroughs or districts can be targeted by the strategy, although because window-advertising reduces costs to the minimum, there is good reason to circulate the message as widely as possible.

6.3.3 School-entry health check-ups for 4–5s

Health check-ups are available for all children during the first year of primary school, although these are only carried out with parental consent. There are three core areas of health checked: growth, hearing and vision.[59] There is no specific requirement for immunisation status to be ascertained nor referral made if the child is behind with their vaccinations.

We recommend that the identification of immunisation status becomes part of the core concerns of the School Entry Health Check, even if this still allows parents to refuse to pass on information, or refuse the option of vaccination catch-up. The nurse can thereby facilitate:

- dissemination of information on the importance of child immunisation (pre-school booster and MMR second dose included)

- updating of GP-CHIS information systems

- referral back to GP for catch-up

- scheduling of immunisation on site, where this is provided by school nursing team

The uptake of DTaP/IPV booster and MMR second dose is generally much lower than the vaccinations for 0–2s. Reasons for lower uptake include the perception among some that boosters and second vaccinations are not always necessary; increased work commitments of parents (by the time the child reaches school age); and the lack of information received prior to invitation to pre-school vaccinations (as compared with the 0-2 programme).[60]

By making the assessment of immunisation status a core component of the School Entry Health Check, the immunisation programme has much greater chance of catching children who are behind in their vaccinations – before they become even more 'hard to reach'.

---

59. http://www.nhs.uk/Livewell/Screening/Pages/Checkschildhood.aspx

60. Tickner S, Leman PJ, Woodcock A. NCBI, 2010. Parents' views about pre-school immunization: an interview study in southern England. Available: http://www.ncbi.nlm.nih.gov/pubmed/19961504

More generally, it is important to seize any 'unscheduled' opportunity for the checking of immunisation status, through contact with midwives, health visitors, GPs or children's centres. Every clinical contact presents an opportunity to reduce health inequalities.

Recommendation	Action to be taken by:
20. The assessment of immunisation status needs to become a core area of the School Entry Health Check for all children. Nurses need to take this opportunity to promote the importance of vaccination and help arrange catch-up where necessary.	PHE LA Public Health

6.3.4 Reaching vaccine-hesitant communities

The relationship between ethnicity and immunisation uptake is recognised as complex, since key determinants include socio-economic factors, religious belief, opinions of community leaders, education, experience from abroad and the process of migration.

But where minority ethnic groups are demonstrably vaccine-resistant or hard to reach, different strategies are sometimes required at the local level to communicate the benefits of immunisation and enable access. The challenge is finding the right intervention with the right business case.

With NHS England now responsible for funding immunisation strategies, tailored interventions at the local level will be undertaken through the Screening and Immunisation Team, who collaborate closely with NHS England Area Teams and local public health.

Variations in local practice may mean additional resources are required on a short-term basis to increase immunisation uptake.

NICE

Immunisation information leaflets in different languages should be available from GP practices and children's centres (appropriate to population needs),[61] although not all members of the minority community may be literate. Information leaflets are also restricted in terms of registering the sometimes complex interactions within the ethnic community itself, or the relationship between the ethnic community and wider community.[62]

Face-to-face interventions require the building of trust and often bilingual competence on the side of the health worker. Strategies to increase uptake may therefore necessitate recruitment from the minority community itself. The London borough of Brent took this approach, commissioning a Somalian key worker to champion immunisation within the local Somalian community. The borough considered the strategy an important lever of increased uptake.[63]

Tower Hamlets, probably home to the largest Somali community in London, chose to set up an educational workshop for Somali advocates and community leaders to dispel the myth of that MMR vaccination causes autism. This was followed by five community workshops, facilitated by a Somali advocate, for Somali parents to discuss their concerns about immunisation and understand the reasons for the MMR vaccination.[64]

61. Public immunisation information in translation is also available from the Health Protection Agency. See: www.hpa.org.uk/MigrantHealthGuide/HealthTopics/InfectiousDiseases/Immunisation/#pat_info
62. For example, see: International Organisation for Migration, 2006. Somali Regions: Mapping exercise, London.
63. 2020health interview with Brent Teaching representative: August 2013
64. Tower Hamlets Joint Strategic Needs Assessment 2010-2011

Another London borough we spoke with was attempting to identify partners from its ethnic minority community who could provide personal testimony about the serious impact of communicable disease. It was thought this would help bring the message 'home' to the hard-to-reach population much more effectively than leaflets or posters. This strategy could be considered for both ethnic minority and traveller communities.

Recommendation	Action to be taken by:
21. NHS England, working with local Public Health, should consider recruiting key workers (such as community health trainers) from the minority community to act as trusted immunisation champions. Such community health workers could operate at an area-wide level if necessary.	NHS England LA Public Health
22. Local strategies may benefit from the engagement of faith group leaders (and more widely religious councils) to help promote the safety and acceptability of vaccines, especially where there is concern expressed around porcine ingredients.	LA Public Health

6.3.5 Text immunisation reminders

Email and SMS messaging are already used within the NHS to alert patients about upcoming appointments. General practice is catching on, with many across England using SMS texting (often in addition to email) as an efficient and cost-effective way to send out notifications and reminders.[65] Available in different language templates, SMS reminders have been seen to reduce DNAs at some GP practices by nearly 50%.[66] Texting services, in particular, present considerable potential for the Childhood Immunisation Programme, for appointment call, confirmation and reminders, also for recall messages if appointments are missed.

We introduced internet appointment booking and auto-text patient reminders and found this greatly [reduced] DNAs.

The Kakoty Practice, Barnsley

There is evidence that text messaging is an effective way of engaging with hard to reach patients;[67] if individuals are likely to possess any technology, this will more often than not be a mobile phone.[68] 92% of UK adults possess a mobile phone, and usage among those with lower incomes or the unemployed (DE group) is above 80%.[69]

The [texting] system has been a huge help, it has made it a lot easier to target parents asking them to call the surgery to book an appointment for their child's vaccination.

Hambleden Clinic, Southwark

65. www.mjog.com/products-services/mjog-for-gp-practices/health-awareness-campaign-messages/
66. www.practicemanagement.org.uk/uploads/access_guide/090702__improving_access_responding_to_patients_final.pdf
67. ibid
68. Ofcom, 'Adult media use and attitudes', March 2012
69. http://www.newmediatrendwatch.com/markets-by-country/18-uk/154-mobile-devices

In terms of access to parents, running costs, and the timing of reminders, text messaging is extremely efficient and some practices have recorded notable financial benefits. Connecting for Health provides an example of a GP practice in Ayrshire, whose text messaging reduced their mail-out for flu jabs and other vaccinations by 50%. Accounting for staff hours, postage and paper, the annual saving to the practice was calculated at £2,230.[70]

Costs of the SMS service vary and there is a range of private 'mobile health' providers already working with the NHS. Connecting for Health's secure NHSmail system (SMS and email) is free for GP practices to use.[71]

For the CIP, automated text and email messaging appears to be a cheap and efficient way of increasing uptake. While the NHS encourages ground-level adoption of SMS texting systems, Screening and Immunisation teams need to be knowledgeable about the potential of the technology and actively promoting its use among GP Practices.

Recommendation	Action to be taken by:
23. The use of text technology needs to be actively promoted among General Practice, so to facilitate efficient appointment call and timely reminders, reducing both paperwork and DNA rates.	Screening and Immunisation Teams CCGs

70. www.connectingforhealth.nhs.uk/systemsandservices/nhsmail/about/benefits/sms_benefits.pdf
71. http://www.connectingforhealth.nhs.uk/systemsandservices/nhsmail/about

7. Conclusion

The recent achievements of the Childhood Immunisation Programme, evidenced by increased uptake since 2008 in most areas of the country, might lead some to think that the programme should just stay its course to see yet further success. But new NHS commissioning structures, instituted April 2013, have themselves forced a rethink of how the CIP is funded, supported and scrutinised; they have also brought an opportunity to consider how the system might achieve greater equity with a more intelligent use of resources.

The system is still settling down and it is too early to assess the effectiveness of the new CIP architecture. But at the same time swift action is needed to bring greater stability to the reformed CIP. The DH has to recognise the enormous variance of CIP support structures currently in place across England. In part, there is variance because there is a lack of protocol or there is confusion. In a few cases we found support being delivered non-commissioned. Some interviewees told us that they were providing non-commissioned support because they could not bear to see their hard work of recent years undermined by present confusion within the CIP.

These support structures include immunisation training and advice pathways. The DH and NHS England need to make clear as to who is responsible for the funding immunisation training, while local Public Health has a duty to establish immunisation advice pathways for their providers (General Practice nurses and community nurses). These are matters of the utmost urgency.

Understaffing in Public Health screening and immunisation (area) teams is also a pressing concern, not least because such teams are a vital agency of strategic support and planning at the local level. Public Health England needs to gear up its efforts to recruit staff and fill vacant posts: the CIP will not function efficiently without them.

Other challenges remain largely the same as they were pre-reforms. The CIP should be striving for higher uptake and reduced inequalities: as the measles outbreak of 2012/13 confirmed, sub-95% uptake represents system failure. Much attention was focused on the situation in Wales, although England itself had 1,386 confirmed cases from January to August 2013, with hospitalisations standing at 294 (21% of total).[72] The data show the highest concentration of cases in the North East and North West, regions of generally higher uptake than the rest of England.

It is important to recognise that even if a Local Authority can claim 95% uptake or more, this does not necessarily guarantee herd immunity for the whole locality. At the district level there may be significant variation: an LA may find most districts with above 95% uptake and a minority (often the more deprived areas) below 90%. Thus a nursery or school situated in a district of low uptake will contain a disease-susceptible population. It is important that Public Health and Area Teams scrutinise COVER figures at the district level and take appropriate measures to combat inequalities.

There is a real opportunity for NHS England Area Teams, with support from screening and immunisation teams, to consider cost-effective strategies at not just the local level but also the area level. There may not be a business case for a dedicated immunisation team or mobile unit to work within the geographical reaches of a single Local Authority; but Area Teams, now as the commissioners of immunisation services, are well placed to consider the area-wide deployment of supporting staff or teams.

---

72. http://www.hpa.org.uk/hpr/archives/2013/hpr4013.pdf

London boroughs could well benefit from examining the success of Tower Hamlets, whose strategic approach has included LES payments to General Practice on a network basis to attain 95% uptake targets. Their high uptake has also relied on strong local leadership, fully interoperable CHIS and GP systems, routine data cleansing, advice to practice managers on call and recall, and targeted MMR information campaigns working alongside Somali community leaders.

In terms of policy amendments, it would be valuable to see changes to the Directed Enhanced Service (DES) structure. Rewarding GPs for hitting 70% uptake is tantamount to rewarding failure. It is surely time to raise the lower target from 70% to 80%. We also recommend a three-tier DES structure, retaining a 90% target, but also introducing a 95% target, with the relative financial rewards changing to 1 (80%): 2.5 (90%): 3.5 (95%). The raising of the lower threshold and the slight reduction on the 90% reward would help finance the new 95% target.

It is also time to bring DES payments into alignment with COVER. The current system allows financial rewards for General Practice even where immunisation is given too late for inclusion in the COVER schedule; GP targets are therefore misaligned with those of Public Health England – and indeed the World Health Organisation. DES payments need to derive from data held on the Child Health Information System (CHIS), thus incentivising timely immunisation and reporting by General Practice.

Recent developments in Wales

In both interviews and at the September workshop opinion was sought on a proposal to enable the barring of unvaccinated children from school or pre-school setting on the occasion (and for the duration) of an outbreak. Feedback was mixed. However, Public Health Wales (PHW) has very recently recommended such a measure, stating that 'where necessary this should be backed by a formal request to co-operate under public health law'.[73] This policy should be debated in England. Adopting the PHW-recommended policy could help raise awareness among parents as to the importance of immunisation. Crucially, the policy implies that while parents can still choose not to have their child vaccinated, their decision must not in any way compromise the physical and educational welfare of other children.

Data flow and accuracy is an often discussed concern of the CIP. NHS England is currently charged with the commissioning of Child Health Immunisation Systems, although this responsibility is expected to pass to local authorities in 2015. NHS England needs to work closely with local Public Health to ensure that progress continues in this vital area, notwithstanding the imminent process of handover. Interoperable CHIS and GP systems may be some way off, but a move toward semi-automated systems via third party software must be a priority for Child Health Departments who are currently hampered by time-intensive manual data processing.

Finally, it would be immensely valuable to see Local Public Health and the DH increasing the dissemination of learning (and materials) around immunisation strategies, whether this derives from ground-level innovation, catch-up campaigns or immunisation awareness schemes. There is a dearth of such information published in the public domain. Details of one of the most interesting and cost-effective catch-up strategies we

---

73. Outbreak of Measles in Wales Nov 2012 – July 2013. Report of the agencies which responded to the Outbreak (Abertawe Bro Morgannwg University Health Board, Powys Health Board, Hywel Dda Health Board and Public Health Wales) October 2013. Report available from: http://www.wales.nhs.uk/sitesplus/888/news/29688

7. Conclusion

found, highlighted in Section 6.3.1 (Halton, North West England, 2008), is currently available only through subscription to a Texas-based bioscience journal. Mobile immunisation unit interventions, such as Hackney's 'Spotty Bus' campaign of 2007, are also underreported. Public Health England needs to ensure routine qualitative and quantitative analyses of such interventions and make materials and learning readily accessible online.

At the September workshop confidence was expressed in continued CIP success amid the NHS reforms and reorganisation. That confidence was challenged by others, who believe the CIP to be currently destabilised by changes to its commissioning and support architecture. Most interviewees expressed similar concerns. The COVER statistics will no doubt reveal the truth over the coming months.

It is hoped readers will have found this report a valuable source of support and encouragement – especially immunisation providers, public health and NHS staff who have in recent years aspired so commendably and successfully to protect the health and wellbeing of our nation's children.

Appendix A: List of interviewees, workshop attendees and steering group members

Interviewees

Name	Position	Organisation
Ike Anya	Deputy director of Public Health	Westminster
Nicki Banyard	Imms Specialist Nurse	Kensington and Chelsea
Luise Dawson	Public Health Nurse	Tower Hamlets
Jose Figueroa	Deputy Director of Public Health, lead on immunisations	Hackney
Dr Reeta Gupta	Consultant Paediatrician	Brent
Elizabeth Hunt	Immunisation Specialist Nurse	Hillingdon
Pauline Macdonald	Nurse Consultant, communicable disease	Public Health, Dudley Metropolitan Council
Carol McCalla	Operational Manager, immunisation team	Ealing NHS Trust
Alison Miller	Public health Principal for infant and maternal health.	Croydon
Andrew J. Pollard	Professor of Paediatric Infection and Immunity / Director of the Oxford Vaccine Centre	Department of Paediatrics / Oxford Vaccine Centre at Oxford University.
Fiona Print	Independent Immunisation	
Andrew Ridley	Advisor	North and East London Commissioning Support Unit
Debbie Saban	Managing Director Screening and Immunisation	Essex Area Team
Stefan Studnik	Manager Consultant Paediatrician	Westminster

Informal (phone/email) contact with immunisation support and/or providers

South Tyneside, Walsall, Havering, Islington, Enfield, Sutton & Merton

Appendix A: List of interviewees, workshop attendees and steering group members

Workshop attendees

Name	Position	Organisation
Dr Sarah Wollaston MP	Member	Health Select Committee
Judith Ashon	Health Visitor Team Leader	St. Charles Family Centre, Central London Community Healthcare NHS Trust
Nicky Banyard	Immunisation Lead	Central London Community Healthcare NHS Trust
Gail Beer	Director of Operations	2020health
Helen Donovan	Public Health Adviser	Royal College of Nursing
Dr Yvonne Doyle	Regional Director, London	Public Health England
Dr David Elliman	Immunisation Representative	Royal College of Paediatrics and Child Health
Dr Alison Frater	Head of Public Health, Military and Offender Commissioning	NHS England (London)
Elizabeth Hunt	Immunisation Specialist Nurse	Central and North West London NHS Foundation Trust
Dr Saul Faust	Reader in Paediatric Immunology and Infectious Diseases	NIHR Wellcome Trust Clinical Research Facility, University of Southampton
Dr David Low	Clinical Informatics Advisor	NHS England
Dr Mary Malone	Programme Leader PostgraduateDiploma (PGDip) Specialist Community Nursing	Florence Nightingale School of Nursing and Midwifery
Julia Manning	Chief Executive	2020health
Daniel Moulin	Director	Sitekit Apps
Dr Simon Nadel	Consultant in Paediatric Intensive Care	St Mary's Hospital and Imperial College London
Dr Kay Nolan	Associate Director, Centre for Public Health	NICE
Katie Panton	UK Government Affairs & Policy	Pfizer (observing)
Jon Paxman	Senior Researcher and CIP Project Lead	2020health

Workshop attendees (continued)

Name	Position	Organisation
Shahida Rasul	Market Development Manager	Pfizer (observing)
Julie Roberts	Team Leader, School Nurse	Stafford and Stone Districts
Dr Lynn Sayer	Programme Leader SCPHN: Health Visiting & School Nursing	Florence Nightingale School of Nursing and Midwifery
Belinda Shear	Universal Services Manager	Sutton and Merton Community Services Manager

Steering Group

Name	Position	Organisation
Gail Beer	Director of Operations	2020health
Michael Corr	Immunisation Clinical Coordinator	Lewisham and Greenwich NHS Trust
Helen Donovan	Public Health Advisor	Royal College of Nursing
Rachel Flowers	Director of Public Health	Public Health Newham
Jon Paxman	Senior Researcher	2020health
Fiona Smith	Adviser in Paediatric Nursing	Royal College of Nursing
Dr Simon Nadel	Consultant in Paediatric Intensive Care	St Mary's Hospital and Imperial College London

Appendix B:
Wales measles outbreak data

The following data, sourced from Public Health Wales, reveals the dangers of sub-optimal uptake of the MMR vaccine. Uptake around 90% still leaves unvaccinated children highly exposed to infection: herd immunity requires at least 95% coverage, which must be sustained year on year. It is interesting to note that Cardiff saw very few notifications, while Swansea (which has in recent years achieved higher average uptake than Cardiff) hosted the worst of the outbreak. The data should provide a clear warning against complacency.

Data presented does not represent laboratory confirmed cases, rather 'notifications of measles reported to Public Health Wales by doctors who have diagnosed a patient with having measles from clinical symptoms.' [74] The effectiveness of the MMR vaccine has been highlighted by PH Wales. Data as of 26 April 2013 showed less than 10 laboratory confirmed cases of measles among MMR-vaccinated children. PHW conclude: 'This emerging data suggests that in the outbreak area one dose of MMR vaccine protects against measles in more than 95 out of every 100 vaccinated, and two doses protects in around 99 out of every 100 vaccinated.' [75]

74. http://www.wales.nhs.uk/sitesplus/888/page/66389#d Accessed 26.11.2013
75. ibid

Number of notifications of measles in Wales in selected
Local Authorities during outbreak period:
1 November 2012 – 03 July 2013

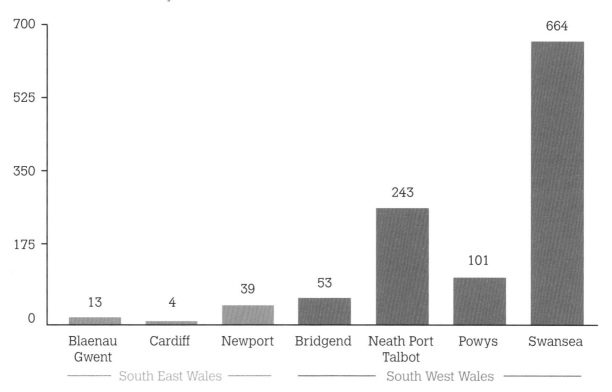

Notifications of measles in Wales (all regions) by age:
1 November 2012 – 03 July 2013

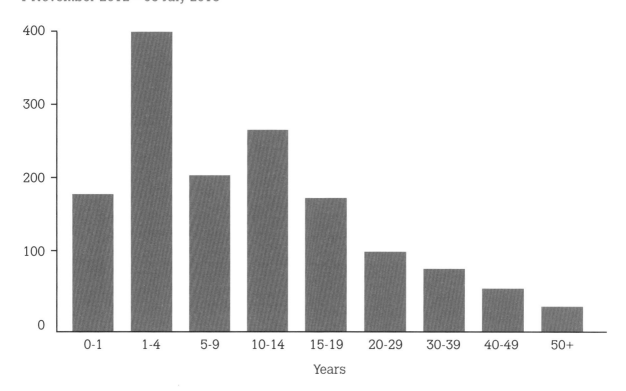

Appendix B:
Wales measles outbreak data

Percentage uptake of MMR Vaccine by 24 months in selected
Local Authorities in Wales from 2007/08 to 2012/13

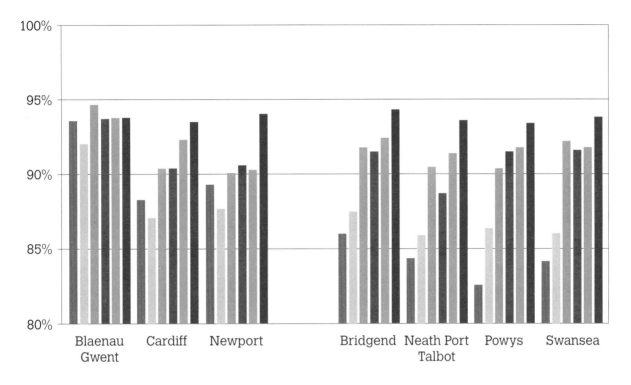

Percentage uptake of MMR Vaccine by 5 years in selected
Local Authorities in Wales from 2007/08 to 2012/13

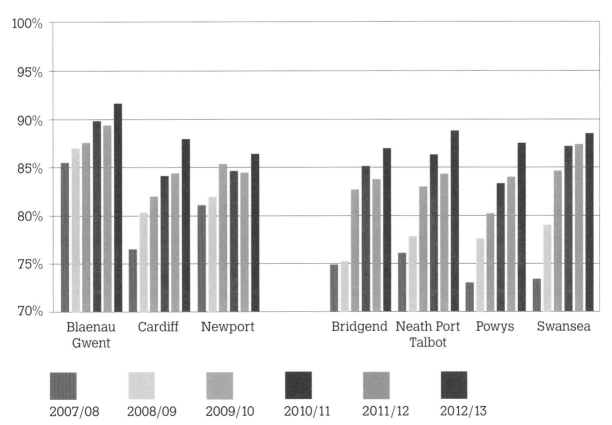

2007/08   2008/09   2009/10   2010/11   2011/12   2012/13

Appendix C:
Unvaccinated Children

Counterpart to Table 3a (Section 3). Children totals at 24 months & 5 years,
with approximate number not fully immunised in selected vaccinations;
selected areas in England: 2012–13.

SHA/PCTs	Total number of Children aged 2 (000s)	N / % not immunised at 24 months			Total number of children aged 5 (000s)	N / % not immunised at 5th birthday	
		DTaP/ IPV/Hib	MMR 1st dose	Hib/MenC booster		DTaP/ IPV booster	MMR 1st and 2nd dose
England	689,447	25,520 / 3.7%	52,933 / 7.7%	50,612 / 7.3%	672,445	74,307 / 11.1%	82,586 / 12.3%
North East	30,862	672 / 2.2%	1,824 / 5.5%	1,394 / 4.5%	29,958	2,093 / 7%	2,496 / 8.3%
South Tyneside	1,725	18 / 1%	30 / 3.4%	43 / 2.5%	1,623	81 / 5%	113 / 7%
Hartlepool	1,144	55 / 4.8%	124 / 10.8%	106 / 9.3%	1,185	46 / 3.9%	155 / 3.1%
North West	87,717	2,266 / 2.6%	4,459 / 5.1%	4,449 / 5.1%	86,455	7 518 / 8.7%	8059 / 8.4%
Salford	3,372	35 / 1%	54 / 1.6%	57 / 1.7%	3,029	80 / 2.6%	91 / 3%
Manchester	7,241	267 / 3.7%	531 / 7.3%	630 / 8.7%	6,929	6,090 / 5.2%	6,043 / 12.8%
West Midlands	71,613	2,463 / 3.4%	5,200 / 7.3%	5,735 / 8%	69,267	7,329 / 10.6%	8,401 / 12.1%
Walsall Teaching	3,385	42 / 1.2%	102 / 3%	106 / 3.1%	3,028	101 / 3.4%	5% / 150
Birmingham East & North	6,698	482 / 1.2%	983 / 4.7%	1,156 / 17.3%	6,260	1,159 / 18.5%	1,280 / 20.4%
London	130,386	8,374 / 6.4%	16,770 / 12.9%	16,494 / 12.7%	123,053	24,747/ 20.1%	23,665 / 19.2%
Tower Hamlets	4,235	115 / 2.7%	263 / 6.2%	236 / 5.6%	3,671	206 / 5.6	241 / 6.6%
Newham	6,411	576 / 9%	1,143 / 17.8%	1,152 / 18%	6,201	1,992 / 32.1%	1,744 / 28.1
Westminster*	2,766	502 / 18.1%	625 / 22.6%	635 / 23%	2,392	560 / 23.4%	589 / 24.6%
South East Coast	54,827	2,743 / 5%	4,661 / 8.5%	4,625 / 8.4%	54,197	5,071 / 9.4%	7,644 / 14.1%
Eastern & Coastal Kent	8,835	212 / 2.4%	464 / 5.3%	472 / 5.3%	8,610	527 / 6.1%	692 / 8%
Surrey	15,432	1,636 / 10.6%	2,535 / 16.4%	2,498 / 16.4%	15,624	2,029 / 13%	3,694 / 23.6%

* Uptake may be higher than reported due to possible lack of systematic reporting of immunisation delivered by private practice.